NANCY FRIDAY

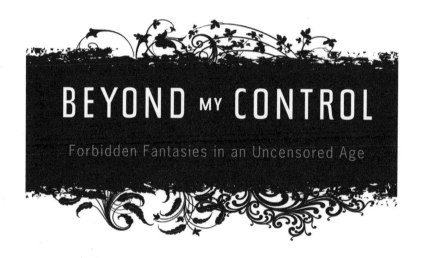

BEYOND MY CONTROL

Forbidden Fantasies in an Uncensored Age

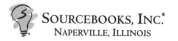

SOURCEBOOKS, INC.®
NAPERVILLE, ILLINOIS

Special thanks to Eric Houston for his editorial assistance.

Published by Sourcebooks, Inc.
P.O. Box 4410, Naperville, Illinois 60567-4410
(630) 961-3900
Fax: (630) 961-2168
www.sourcebooks.com

Library of Congress Cataloging-in-Publication Data

Friday, Nancy.
  Beyond my control : forbidden fantasies in an uncensored age / Nancy
Friday.
     p. cm.
  1. Sexual fantasies. 2. Paraphilias. I. Title.
  HQ71.F75 2009
  306.77--dc22

                                            2008049271

       Printed and bound in the United States of America
             BG 10 9 8 7 6 5 4 3 2 1

FOR BOB THIXTON,

The best agent and, oh yes, friend! a writer could have.

ALSO BY NANCY FRIDAY

My Secret Garden
Forbidden Flowers
My Mother, My Self
Men in Love
Jealousy
Women on Top
The Power of Beauty (Our Looks / Our Lives)

CONTENTS

AUTHOR TO READER
Still My Secret Garden

Over thirty-five years ago, I called it *My Secret Garden* because collecting fantasies was like listening to women whispering in my ear. I was hearing their deepest erotic secrets—in many cases, desires they had not even told themselves until then. Still today, many women and men finish by saying, "Thank you for letting me tell you."

I know precisely what they mean. There is something about putting sex into writing, almost as if we are taking it to the next level of reality, getting closer and closer to the flame. At the same time, it is emboldening, as in: "This is who I am—who I really am! And look…the sky hasn't fallen, I haven't been ostracized from the family, and I feel more complete, whole, part of the human race."

Yes, I do believe that for many of us, accepting our erotic reveries opens a new consciousness in our lives. We don't have to act on the fantasies to feel this way. Some, fully realized, would become nightmares. Nor share them with our partners. Often, kept from them, they can be even more emboldening. It is thrilling just to own the creativity of our sexual imagination. Just as learning to drive opens new paths—emotionally as well as physically—so do our private sexual thoughts, at any age, take us on ever-new trips, as doors open and horizons broaden.

We like to think that we are formed by what we choose to take in, while from the day we were born, we have been absorbing the opinions of the people on whom we are dependent. Our caretakers' opinions (often unspoken) of our body are woven into our self-image. Later, changes that we choose to make will be in opposition to theirs.

Our tiny hand goes between our legs because it feels good and, yes, because it is our body. So, there we are, not even able to use adverbs, and the giants of the nursery are laying down lifelong prejudices. They say, "No, no, darling…" and remove our hand from that sweet crevice. We won't remember it or a dozen other repeated sounds and actions that over time hammer home *their* opinions of *our* genitals.

So often our devoted caretakers would deny any role in turning us away from our sexual parts, so automatic and unthinking were their intentions. If accused in court of crippling someone's sexual self-esteem, they would look askance.

By the time we choose a sexual mate, have a certificate of marriage, or become economically independent, we will also have a private stash of erotic fantasies, stored since adolescence, helping us get past the negative opinions of other people regarding *our* sexual parts. Now, when our mind and body want to boost us up, up, and away into orgasm, we call upon these fantasies to do their magic.

Our response to the thrill of sexual feeling in adolescence is electric. It is so sweet, so winning, yes, so natural, that it is hard to ally it with the negative experience long ago in the nursery. This is something new and beautiful, what we feel in one another's arms at adolescence. That so many young girls get pregnant when they have been raised never to let a lad anywhere near that forbidden fertile ground until the appropriate moment speaks of the beauty of erotic rapture—something the girl might understand and deal with had she been taught to respect "that place." But raised on distaste and abhorrence of her genitals, the girl eagerly hands herself over to the boy/man and crowns him a Prince for loving that "unspeakable" core of herself.

Before the sexual revolution of the twentieth century, most women denied their erotic fantasies. Young adults today find that hard to believe. Where did these forbidden, unacceptable fantasies go after they were enjoyed, these rich erotic thoughts that accompanied our sex? Can the mind actually entertain a sexual fantasy during intercourse or masturbation and then erase it post-orgasm?

I thought I'd heard everything with regard to my favorite subject until I received this missive in 2002 from a twenty-three-year-old English woman:

"Dear Nancy, I always thought it was only famous, rich, successful—as in some way privileged women—who had sexual fantasies. Finding out that so many ORDINARY WOMEN [her caps] enjoy sex so much is a fantastic thing to know. It makes me feel so much better to realize that anyone can have a great sex life."

Such a funny, sweet thought makes me want to put my arm around the dear girl and welcome her into the club.

But, of course, masturbation only came onto the scene, front and center, in the last thirty years. Certainly, some women masturbated but not in the epidemic proportions we do today. (Hah! Fun to imagine an "epidemic" of women masturbating; the headlines in the newspapers: "All traffic comes to a halt as women across the world masturbate for world peace!")

One thing I've learned absolutely is that forbidden sex gets us higher faster. We may love our mate, but love and sex are separate, different, and there is no denying the thrill of stolen sex, in fantasy and in reality. The more forbidden, the more intense the orgasm. And if the man inside us isn't off-limits, well, then, within the secret room of our imagination, we envision someone who is. Not only is the man off-limits but so is the locale where we do the dirty deed—the bus, a train, behind the cereal section in the supermarket, under the table in the restaurant, or perhaps with the handsome stranger beside us in an airplane. We wait until the movie begins, the lights lower, and the blanket, hopefully still provided by the flight attendant, can shield him as he slips between our legs and applies his hands, his mouth, his considerable talent to bring us to orgasm.

We can't afford to actually have sex with the man next door with whom our husband plays golf, but when we want to climb to orgasm, we imagine him breathing heavily in our ear during the dance, and we two disappear when no one is looking. In seconds, we're secluded or—more dangerous and exciting—we take a terrible chance of getting caught and pull him down upon us in the guest room. Quick, quick! His penis is inside us, it no longer matters if we're found, so close are we to orgasm.

Could Adam and Eve resist the apple? Do we really believe it was all about an apple? There is no way to make the safe sex of marriage as exciting as the forbidden. We salt and pepper sex with our legal mate, imagining forbidden men in forbidden places.

Is it any wonder pain, force, verbal abuse are often attached to our real sex, maybe something slight like the bite on the nipple, the added thrust of the penis, abusive words: "You are a bad little bitch, and Daddy's going to punish you," our lover says playfully. "Harder! Deeper!" we cry out when his penis is inside us, so deep we get the pleasure and the pain confused.

Why do we seek a certain form of intimacy or avoid it? Whatever "fits" may have its roots in a time before we can remember.

Money, too, is part of the sexual drama because it symbolizes undeniable power. Men and women have always been afraid of each other. Why do you think at some point most men have paid for sex? It was a high price, but the alternative would have meant never getting away from the first woman who controlled his life totally. Oh, yes, he loved her, but you know as well as I that the stories of guys who never get away from their mothers are either comic or tragic.

"Powder me, powder me!" a former lover cried out when I was crouched between his legs, his cock in my mouth.

Where did that come from? I asked myself and answered: Hadn't I interviewed him in our early days together? His early memory of days with his mom had to do with her weeping when she bathed him because his father was away in the war. And he, only a very little boy, would say to her, "But I'm here, Mommy!" To which she would reply, sadly, "You are not enough."

She got him coming and going, so to speak. By the time he ended up in my bed, he was a mass of contradictions, wanting to be babied and on top. But he is not alone in his sexual split. Most men solve the Madonna/whore dilemma by making their wives the safe haven (calling the wife "mother") and looking for forbidden sex with "bad" women.

A comfortably married woman tells me: "Before marriage, we were more adventurous. (Mild bondage, lots of head, etc.) After marriage, my husband would pull me up when I'd go down on him—like, now that I was his wife, it was somehow 'dirty.'"

The above may be more true of traditional men and women—meaning pre-feminism—than of couples today where both work outside the home. Nothing has changed women more from the stereotypical housewife who took care of home and nurtured children than women's entry into the workplace. There is nothing like a weekly salary, the independence that comes with paying the rent and buying groceries, even if the money barely covers costs, to dispel the self-image of "little girl." Put another way, depending on someone else for the roof over your head and food on the table puts a big dent in creative sex. At least, this is what I've come to believe. It's not necessarily conscious, thought-out reasoning; it just goes with the territory: "I pay my own way. I want sex my own way." If orgasm is the state of letting go, I can let go because I'm in charge of me.

For over thirty years, I've been writing about eros, love, jealousy, beauty, envy, all subjects that invariably lead back to childhood. Nothing is more immutable than what happened in those years when we had no power at all. What we did have was total *absorption*. We couldn't control what to take in or leave out. Unable to feed or clothe ourselves, totally dependent on others, they left their prints all over us.

The 1970s, that very special era in which *My Secret Garden* was written, possess continued relevance. They were profoundly influential years, not just regarding sex but all forms of behavior. The top of the list is an army of women who moved out of the home and into every sphere and endeavor that men had owned up to then.

The revolutionary shift in the fundamental truths of what men and women were, how they saw themselves, and what work defined them gave me permission to write about something that had clearly been on my mind and was part of my own sexuality. I loved original work and always had sexual fantasies. As I've noted before, when I approached several eminent therapists and psychoanalysts and asked their opinion of my research, I was repeatedly told: "Women do not have sexual fantasies. Men do."

I was confused but not discouraged. I had collected a variety of women's erotic daydreams. We were a new world of sisters, a secret society, about to go public. And if a woman didn't initially know what a sexual fantasy was, I'd simply tell her my own and the curtains would part. "Oh, is *that* a sexual fantasy!? Sure, I've had those." She'd had them for years, used them to reach orgasm, and then, being a "good girl," swallowed the forbidden thought.

So, here we are, dear friends, a new century, a new age of equality—and what is the overwhelming theme of fantasy in this book, for both men and women? *Domination*. Not dominating but *being dominated*. Relinquishing power in a world that offers so much.

Women's worlds used to be limited by Do's and Don'ts. Even we intelligent, danger-loving girls *had* fantasies but didn't own them. We secretly longed for a guy from the wrong side of the tracks. We enjoyed him but often didn't tell the other girls. His "forbiddenness" made our secret thoughts even that much more thrilling.

This book is the first in which I'm including both men's and women's fantasies. In a world where we are able to duplicate one another's jobs, clothes, almost everything in the dance of life, I thought it might be interesting to see where we run parallel in erotic dreams. Do women now imagine themselves seducing their favorite sex objects and do men dream of being taken, often against their will?

Has the Internet leveled the playing field? Can the virtuous woman easily change her identity and take to bed a different stranger every night or anonymously chat online, satisfying both their fantasies?

We lie, pretend, often unaware. Riddled with fear, jealousy, insecurity, who has not projected confidence? To some degree, we are the serial killer personifying the pillar of the community. How much more has the Internet opened the door to our fantasy selves—a cyber world of infinite possibilities? Reese, a sixty-five-year-old gay man, admits that "through the miracle of the Internet, I am now a super-hot eighteen-year-old blonde cheerleader."

It is hard to believe there ever was a time when we weren't fully aware of our erotic reveries. But sexual freedom is never fully won. When *My Secret Garden* was published in 1973, *Ms.* magazine wrote that "Friday is no feminist," and *Cosmopolitan*'s favorite male psychoanalyst echoed—emphasizing again—"Men have sexual fantasies; women do not." Although this was the past, it's wise to remember that sexual repression never sleeps. Never take sexual freedom for granted.

Eventually, the pendulum may swing back. It always has. How short a time it's been that women came to own their erotic fantasies. Thirty, forty years, a drop in the bucket.

Don't presume that these dark days are behind us; so powerful is the image of the out-of-control orgasmic woman that it turns off many people, scares both women and men. We may put a woman in the White House but not a woman who comes across as powerfully sexual.

I believe that sexual fantasy is a natural, healthy part of us, an evolved dimension used to aid our pleasure and excitement. Often, it's a necessity for sustaining long-term sexual relations. I remember long ago someone saying dismissively: "I don't need fantasy. My sex life is just fine without it." But fantasies don't have to make up for something that is "missing." They can add extra helium to a balloon that wants to soar. For some of us, the imagery comes unbidden. We close our eyes and let "sex" and "fantasy" join in concert to remove us from the real life that holds us to Earth. Now, here, alone with our lover, the sight, smell, and touch of his body begins to work on us.

The forbidden pleasures, the stolen watermelons in our youth, and the kisses in the parked cars of adolescence—in fantasy, we spread our legs for the stranger who has just blown into town or we imagine the last man who undressed us with his eyes, not our husband, our "legal" mate, no, we may love him, but for orgasm, we need the bad guy, the dark, illicit situation, because that's how we were raised, conditioned, taught to think of the sex we stole.

Over the years, the voices of the men and women in this book have been filed away in my subconscious. Even when printed on the pages of my books, your voices whisper in my ear. I like to keep it that way, our bond, like the tight allegiances of childhood where we told our best friend "everything."

I am ready to dive back into your "confessions"—perhaps not the correct word. But I do get the feeling that while you may begin with a "public" story of your life, I am aware of that special moment when you close the door of whatever room you are in and begin to confide in me what you have never revealed before.

You have been my teachers, my familiars, letting me into your erotic thoughts, private tales many of you say "you've never told anyone before." The first women who came into my secret garden over thirty years ago were breaking the law, saying out loud the thoughts and feelings never before admitted. I often had a sense of looking over their shoulders as they wrote, emboldened to name their thoughts by other women's voices.

Slowly, the chorus of your voices has grown bolder. That so

many of the themes of fantasies in this particular book deal with domination—*being* dominated—has certain logic. The dance between men and women in the modern world has changed. I am speaking of the erotic dance where men once led absolutely. As I've said, women are formidable. We always were. In the past, we simply denied it.

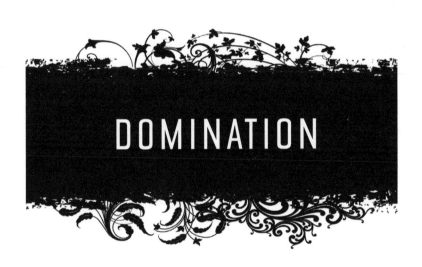

DOMINATION

DOMINATION

Nothing has made me more a traveler in the state of forbidden eros, a lover of danger, than the mystery of my father, whom I never knew, never saw, not even a photo of him, and of whom not a word was ever spoken. Silence and secrecy surrounded him to the degree that "forbidden" became who he was and, by extension, other men too. When people asked in a friendly fashion, "Where is your father, darling?" I'd answer politely, "My daddy's dead."

He wasn't. I found this out at the age of twenty, directly after his death in the mental institute where he had been committed not long after my birth. Given the secrets in my home, I'd become an incurable sleuth, opening every door, especially those marked "Do Not Enter." I'd find a way into neighbors' houses up and down the street, often by way of a cellar door, a screen door left ajar. I was five or six, and ours was a small town populated by kind and gentle people. In such a place, everyone had time for a little girl on a quest, and I never thought twice about following a friendly elderly couple home for a Coca-Cola and a piece of cake nor did they scold me for opening doors and drawers.

I looked everywhere for him, for a trace, a photo, some clue, though I was never aware of my goal. Had someone asked, "What are you looking for?" I'd have answered, "Oh, nothing, just looking." It helped that my town belonged to another era. In retrospect, it seems covered with a sheer layer of magic dust. When I was unable to find even a trace of him, I turned my curiosity to the waterfront. We were on the southern coast, and freighters came and sailed away daily, just a block from our house. I've always seen it as a place lost in time.

My absent father had an influence over me unlike that of anyone else. My pleasure of writing about men, women, sex, forbidden topics, came from him, from my search and eventual need to find in other men what I knew he would have given me. My erotic fantasies of men, my interest in sex as far back as I can remember, all this was heightened by my father, the mystery.

Because the cocktail hour was a staple of life, come six o'clock, our house was a merry place. I would crawl into the lap of a naval officer, inhale the scent of him, light his cigarette, charm him with my song, do a little dance, and pay no attention to my mother's repeated "Leave the gentleman alone, dear." But the gentleman never seemed to mind. How utterly fascinating men were! So relaxed, so easy in their skin. What was their secret, these people in trousers, around whom my mother and all the other women acted differently, all the while pretending they weren't. Something was in the air when men were around, and both men and women looked at one another as though they had a secret. And who better to pick up on this unnamed dance between the grown-ups at the cocktail hour than an overly curious, precocious child?

For me to admit that it made a difference, not having a daddy, that I was sad or that I ever wondered about him was unthinkable. Though no one ever said the word, I knew my role was to protect my mother and not ask. Where did I put my dreams of him when I was little, this constant protector, strong, handsome, kind-hearted with a permanent shoulder for me to rest my head on? The fantasy of being chased by him as he became the "hungry monster" to my gleeful screams of terror, catching me, tickling me, throwing me in the air? When I grew older and a boy held me in his arms, the missing man in my life clicked in. How I loved being held by a boy, his scent, his wanting me, the whole dream state of what I called "love," though it was surely in great part eros.

There are more of us today, fatherless children growing up without a male presence, an atmosphere where we might take in the exciting difference between the sexes. Today, births to unmarried women constitute 36%, reaching a record high, not to mention the near 50% of marriages that end in divorce. Children are sponges, growing, changing, absorbing everything, so much more than adults want to realize. My search for this mysterious man led a search for myself. Had he been present, I undoubtedly would have settled down, married, raised a family, with no consideration to writing about sex.

In the '60s and '70s, the publishing world had thrown open its door to women and was signing us up like recruits. Editors were eager for books on women's lives, interior and exterior. We were like an undiscovered continent. The world finally wanted to know: "What do women want sexually? How does eros feel to a woman inside and out?"

To this day, I am thrilled to have been a part of those halcyon years when we women came out, came alive, discovered the clitoris and our sexual fantasies—to own them. Our sexual independence—knowing that we control and are responsible for our sexual destiny—feeds into all other freedoms.

Knowing that we no longer had to wait for a man to telephone—for him to give us an orgasm—that we could do this for ourselves, and bring him to orgasm, too, was a source of energy to be used in every endeavor of our lives. Owning my sexuality has changed how I walk, talk, and certainly how I write.

The fact remains that in real life and in fantasy, domination remains one of the few forbidden acts that still sexually excites. It is not pain that is wanted—that is reserved for the chapter on S&M—but a powerlessness, a chance to relieve ourselves of all responsibility for the delicious, forbidden sex we crave. We who reach for this kind of imagery in order to let go of the iron self-control that stands in the way of orgasm are wanting a cocktail that "knocks me out beyond my control!"

FANTASIES OF BONDAGE
"Those Ropes Are Too Tight! Thank You!"

Today, many of us reach for erotic scenes that refuse to take "No!" We crave a source of power and restraint—to keep us "grounded" even as we soar. Listen to the voices in this book and hear how early these feelings begin, often from men and women who have never been abused, neglected, or abandoned. Where do the fantasies start? When we are pinned down in our crib, strapped into our high chair, our stroller, the bed where our diapers are changed, our cries for freedom are heard by a loving mother who gazes down on us, gently singing, comforting, but refusing to set us free from our restraints. Or we see an angry mother, frustrated, tormented by our pleas for help, binding us in an attempt to hold her world together. Then, there are the abusive caretakers—people who should never have or be responsible for children. They hit our hands to keep us from struggling for freedom, ignoring, reprimanding our cries as we, in our most helpless state, have to believe she/he loves us, that this is for our own good.

The seeds of our domination fantasies go back to the time when we were helpless, trapped, waiting, longing for a loving guardian. The seeds grow, blossom in whatever direction the earth and nutrients allow. The high school bully forcing us to kiss the ground, the older brother or sister twisting our arms behind our backs, the good-hearted loving father becoming the "hungry monster" to our gleeful screams. Sometimes, we defy those oppressive years to now dominate, to be the all-powerful mother; other times, we long to go back into mother's arms, constrained, gazed at, taken care of.

Not long ago, domination/submission was defined by gender. A fallacy of a male-dominated world. Our biological makeup and countless experiences, nature and nurture, mold us into some degree of both. Why are so many of us inclined to fantasies of domination and submission? Often, the horrific experience of rape is followed by rape fantasies, but why are so many of the fantasies submissive, only now in control, choosing the assailant and circumstances, and others aggressive, now raping the assailant? To both questions, the answer is still unknown.

We don't like to think that small children have sexual feelings. It would require more thought, a deeper involvement in our children's lives—as the bedrock of sexuality is being laid—when we are already overwhelmed by the duties of society and childcare.

Wafting down from orgasm and full of gratitude, I once whispered to my lover, "How did you do that?" He replied, not unkindly, "Nancy, it's all in your head." Thus began my awareness of my own fantasies, such as the dark stranger gazing at me, taking me against my will, forcing me into ecstasy.

I handed over to each man full credit for my rapture. Today, I am still besotted by a man who brings me to orgasmic highs, even though I know it is I who lets him in the gate and leads him up the garden path.

In the fantasies and stories of the brave men and women in this book is a message of how very early sexual feelings—and the theme of erotic reveries—begin. Wheels inside our heads now carry us out of our tight skin, to hold us momentarily in suspense until all the doors open one by one, allowing us to let go.

Karla

Karla is a sixteen-year-old virgin from a liberal family. Her father is a commercial artist and her mother a head librarian. She shares with many of us the fantasy of being taken, of being irresistible.

I am kidnapped by Justin Timberlake, who is a little obsessed with me. Justin takes me to his secluded home in Los Angeles and ties me up in the bathroom and leaves me there while he goes downstairs to record some music. When he returns, he lets me loose on the condition that I don't try to escape or hurt him. I agree. I see that the bed is his destination. It is a huge four-poster with dark blue drapes. I cry out as he ties me to the bed, spread-eagle. He pushes a dildo up my cunt and then leaves. I squirm so that the dildo starts to move inside me. Just as I am about to cum, Justin comes back into the room and takes the dildo out. I start to cry I am so frustrated. He smiles and leans down to kiss me. Then, he starts to lick my pussy, carefully circling my clit and then plunging his tongue deep inside me until I cum, screaming in ecstasy.

I have a few variations on this. One is where my parents insist I get a tutor for history. They choose a stern, forty-something male teacher who happens to look like Viggo Mortensen. Since he's so much older, they feel there's no need for them to stay at home when he is tutoring me. Since I'm already quite good at history to the extent that the tutoring is unnecessary (this actually happened in real life due to parental pressure to excel in school), my tutor decides to teach me about sex instead. I am afraid of him but also curious. He makes me sit on a chair and takes off my top and panties. Then, he ties me to the bed spread-eagle and starts reading from a book about Hitler as a man. As he reads, he puts two of his fingers up my cunt and starts to finger-fuck me.

We hear a woman say in her fantasy: "That big, bad man *forced me* to orgasm. He made me do it." But even in her imagination, she doesn't own up to the depth of her sexual appetite, doesn't want the responsibility. Even in fantasy, she strains against the sexual attention she craves by at first trying to stop the man and then placing the entire burden of being "fucked" on him.

Falling back on the fantasy of being dominated is a desire to take "the control away from me, one way or another." The woman with a crippling fear of rejection often has the fantasy of someone seducing/overwhelming her. In reality, she may be a totally controlling person: "By making him lose control (have an orgasm) even if I don't have an orgasm, *I'm in control.*" In the end, she gets him coming and going (all puns intended).

Scott

Scott, a single white man in his forties, comes from the heartland and says his parents were "from the old school." Sex was never mentioned in his home. He was never hit or sexually abused. His parents kissed, said that they loved each other, but there was an absence of any sign of lovemaking. Do his fantasies of bondage begin in the crib, the memory of longing, waiting? Is the secret exhibitionist in all of us from a time when we were gazed down upon by a stream of adoring large eyes?

I was a typical farm boy growing up. When I was twelve years old, my mother took me to the library and checked out some sex books for me. It was my only education in sex! I played with girls on the street. There were three girls I played a couple of games with on a regular basis. The first game was when the girls would let me cover their mouths with one of my hands and hold their arms behind their backs.

But one night, my parents were gone, and my friends and I were home alone. I don't know what I was thinking, but I stood up and pulled off my T-shirt. They started getting excited. Then, I pulled down my jeans and underwear. They just stared at my penis. I waddled over to the couch and stood there, so each girl could get a good look. They asked me to turn around and show them my butt.

I was married for a while, and my ex-wife was OK in the bedroom but didn't want to add any spice to our sex life until I talked her into tying me up and gagging me. She ordered me to strip completely naked, then ordered me to sit on the chair. She tied each of my ankles to the front legs and tied my wrists with a couple of skinny leather belts. She rolled up a large red bandana and placed it in my mouth and tied it tightly behind my head. Then, she proceeded to get dressed and leave the house. She was going out with a few of her girlfriends. I was bound and gagged to that chair for six hours.

I have many fantasies, but the one that I want to fulfill is to be dominated by a female. I want her to have control of me. I want her to tie me up, gag me, spank me, place clothespins on my nipples, make me worship the ground she walks on.

Why do so many of us, especially men, deny the profound influence of she who carried us inside her body for nine months, only to then care for us until we were able to care for ourselves? We are formed in her emotional image, at least with regard to our ability to love our body, ourselves, and another person.

Why are women so reluctant to own up to their power and influence? Even under patriarchy, men were totally ruled by women growing up, followed by the awesome power of the sexual beauty of the young girls of adolescence. By the time a boy is a young man, he's realized without consciously deciding it that it may be better to marry a quiet girl, pretty, yes, but not a sexually adventurous one who would possibly put him in the role of the betrayed husband.

There are, of course, those men who need to dominate, to feel the reins of power in order to reach orgasm. Stripped of their sexual dominance, in the shadow of the giantess women—who, in some men's eyes, seem to run the world today—these men find orgasm imagining themselves so powerful as to put the woman in her place, where she belongs, beneath him.

Ian

Ian, a middle-aged man from Australia, describes this typical man-on-top domination fantasy, the kind we're used to.

My fantasy comes into play whenever a snarling feminist berates men. In it, I belong to a secret society that kidnaps women and takes them to a specially built prison high in the mountains. The women are trained to become feminine again and enjoy sex with men. They are kept naked at all times. Their training begins by being tied with their arms above their heads while their bodies are slowly massaged with baby oil by the men. We are well aware that pleasure is the best way to condition and so we ensure that all inmates orgasm at each encounter with each one of us.

Demi

In the fantasies of eighteen-year-old Demi, domination by a man empowers her to dominate at the end. Still in school in the (conservative) South, she'd like this fantasy of being asked to the penthouse apartment of her dream lover to actually come true.

I'm pretty vivid in how I see him. He has incredible light brown eyes with the passion of a wildfire, hands of a lumberjack, and an apartment to die for, super modern, like he owns the world. I get there and follow the instructions in an envelope with my name on it. After showering, fixing my hair and makeup, and wearing only high heels, I follow a petal-strewn path to a beautifully set table. He appears wearing a tux. After a candlelit dinner, he takes me into the bedroom. He walks over to the night stand and pulls out a pair of handcuffs. "These are for you," he says. As he handcuffs me to the bedposts, I smile with great anticipation. The sex is so intense, our bodies sound like someone getting whipped. The bed is shaking, and the wealthy neighbors below are complaining, but we don't care. He lifts my legs over my head and goes in deeper, hitting my g-spot. We cum as one. After a few minutes, he unhandcuffs me, and I quickly grab the handcuffs from him and cuff him to the bed. The look of surprise as I take control is all over his face.

When I think of the gulf between boring sex and the kind of wildness we can allow ourselves, it is baffling why so many of us spend so many years living with the former. Do we, like Cara, a beautiful, twenty-six-year-old Latin American woman, put up with the dull sex because it is in keeping with the "good man/ good woman" we are most of the time? Great, orgasmic sex is mind-blowing, out-of-control. For a few moments, we are not ourselves. Floating back down to Earth, post-orgasm, we wonder why we sometimes reserve this extraordinary experience for a near stranger, someone met at a party?

Cara

When I had my first menstrual period, the only thing I remember my mom telling me was that it was really important that I clean myself thoroughly. I know she was only concerned that I not get an infection, but I wonder, was that when I started to feel that the whole process was dirty and I wanted no part of it?

About my sexual life, I have all these ideas and fantasies but don't ever act on them because just the thought of doing so makes me embarrassed. I guess I'm also worried that I would be rejected and laughed at. My parents were divorced when I was five, and we moved far away from my dad. He is not a very motivated person, so I didn't see much of him when I was young. It took me a very long time to realize that I felt abandoned and rejected by him. I think that's where the fear of rejection started. I was also being mentally, and possibly physically and sexually, abused by my mom's boyfriend at the time, so that didn't help. I've slept with about ten men and have only had rare, small orgasms. I've had relationships and casual sex flings, although never one-night stands, and have yet to relax my guard enough to have a screaming orgasm.

I've also picked up this idea that the man's pleasure is more important than mine. That means that I'm putting him in control while I have to stay in control. Is it any wonder that my fantasies center around a man, usually someone I know, staying in control of himself long enough to make me lose it? Someone who ignores my attempts to get him off and concentrates on me?

I have this one fantasy where I'm tied to a bed, and my lover comes in and brushes me with light touches, fleeting, never in the same place twice. He ignores the obvious places and touches me in spots I never knew were erotic. He continues this for hours, ignoring me as I beg him to untie me so I can move, touch him, anything. I can't see what he's doing, what he's touching me with, where he'll touch next, and I'm writhing on the bed. He does this until I have no choice but to cum. Then, he starts over again until I've had so many orgasms, I'm twitching and can't move. After he's done with me, he cuddles me until I fall asleep.

I hope that Cara will find the courage to investigate her full potential in a brave new world. Instead of people laughing, I believe she'll discover that her fantasies are natural, not uncommon, and sought after.

Glory

I'm a thirty-one-year-old woman from Texas and was raised in a sexually free household. I love my body and the potential it creates *for me and for my partner. My body is mine to give. My sexuality is my independence; it is my strength from which my power and lust for life comes.*

My grandma once wrote that as a child I was "confident, determined, not afraid, and eager to learn what the world held." That world for me, I think, unlike other children, started with my body and moved outward. I can remember the intrigue, the fascination with my fingers, my breasts, my vagina, touching my breasts in the bath, caressing myself in bed.

"Mom," I would ask, "Why is my vagina always covered up? Is it bad?"

"No," she would say. "Think of it as your finger—something you should look at and be comfortable with."

My parents, walking from their bedroom to the bathroom naked, playing with each other in the shower, letting my brother and me crawl around in their beds even when they were sleeping with only their skins to the sheets, instilled within me a peace with my body.

I like to touch myself and have for as long as I can remember. However, I have only been reaching orgasm through masturbation since I was a freshman in college. I don't have long sexual fantasies. Mine are all rooted in people I know, people I can actually touch, want to touch, or have touched. It's interesting that all of my fantasies are rooted in reality—I don't usually want my fantasies to remain fantasies. Why do some women fantasize about the impossible and others fantasize about reality? What does this say about each "type" of woman?

My fantasies start with an image of a person, a flash of a familiar face, a smell of a certain man, a sound that recalls someone—and from there, my mind works. My fantasies range from my tying a man up and doing everything in my power to please him, to my taking the part of the "victim," to both of us actively working to satisfy each other. The smells of him. Eyes shut. Relaxed in bed. Licking toes, the tongue moves up the inside of my leg, the hands caress my inner thighs…I want to take those fantasies and make them a reality with that man.

FANTASIES OF WORSHIP
"I Live to Grovel"

With more single moms, boys are being raised without a man in their lives in whom they might see themselves, a person they might choose to emulate or not, a man with influence and power within the family. Can we be surprised that more men than ever automatically reach for the dominatrix?

Families are built upon rules, as in any society. Certainly, there were parental rules regarding sex when we were young and societal rules later on, though breaking them—stopping just short of "going all the way"—carried a thrill that could make up for the guilt.

Historically, mothers enforced the rules. In the most important years of their children's lives, they laid down the "shall-nots"— some fair, some maybe not. Rules can create an atmosphere of safety, mental ropes that keep the child from *"falling off the edge,"* even when the child complains of feeling restricted. By controlling their children's lives through nurture and discipline, they were instilling not just love but fear/anxiety/trepidation should their rules be broken. These were the formative years. In the end, what mattered wasn't that all the rules were obeyed but that they were there, something that you counted on. Even if you disliked them and disobeyed them occasionally, by their very existence, they made you feel safe. They were the constant boundaries against which we fought. Boundaries we now use and break in fantasies to free ourselves to orgasm.

In fantasies of domination, we either enforce these rules/boundaries or submit to them, sometimes pleading, "No, no, please, stop!" other times applauding, worshipping, "Thank you, thank you, Master/Mistress."

The powers of invention have been worn out at the office, and both men and women find that the body lets go, relaxes, and warms up when the mind travels to images of being totally out of control. Jonathan, a married man whose wife is happy with sex once or twice a week, speaks of this yearning. "My fantasy is that when I arrive at the address of my lover, I must be prepared for complete submissiveness, ready to offer my whole mind and body to her, for she will teach me what she likes, and I must obey."

"Forced" to let go of the "manly, man in charge, on top" role he inherited, he gives himself over to orgasm at the hands of a dominating woman.

Henry

Henry, a young interior designer who lives in Chicago, met his current girlfriend online by answering an ad looking for a "sub man."

I was pretty nervous when we first met. I fantasized a long time about being with a hot dominant woman and read lots of ads, but this was the first one I answered. There was something about her authority saying, "I know what's best for you." We exchanged some pictures, and she said she was willing to meet me to see if I was worthy. We met at a bar in her area. It was kind of comforting the way she took control. I felt excited by it. She allowed me to go back with her to her house. When we got there, she said, "Do not look at me unless I give you permission. Now, close your eyes when in my presence, and in the meantime, fix me a drink." When I returned with her drink, she pushed me to the ground and pressed my face to the floor with her foot. She ordered me to undress, and while I did, she unbuttoned her dress from the bottom. She whispered, "Kneel and kiss my cunt." I could feel a dewy drop of precum easing from my prick. I dropped to my knees and felt the increasing warmth of her sex and the convergence of her beautiful strong thighs as I eased my head between her legs.

I've asked her permission to marry her. So far, she hasn't granted it. But I'm still hopeful. I would like to serve her for the rest of my life.

We've found that as one sex changes, the opposite sex adjusts, not necessarily moving in tandem. Certainly, men's erotic fantasies of being dominated by women are more prevalent today than ever. Domination and submission seem to have become a game between men and women, a continuation from the nursery to the office to the bedroom of either sex being submissive or controlling.

Men's sexual arousal, imagining themselves groveling opposite the dominatrix (even after contending with bossy women in the workplace), was no doubt laid down in childhood, when the boy was malleable, soft clay. Many men are still reluctant to interfere with their wife's domain. On some level he is probably afraid of her, too, as he was of his mother.

Men's fantasies of female domination come in all shapes and sizes. Oscar, a Canadian man, twenty-five years old, says, "I have always found women in 'power suits' attractive—even more so than in lingerie." Many men and women write to me about sexual fantasies with authority figures, teachers, bosses, etc.

Sean

Forty-year-old Sean gives me a lighthearted account of being stripped and "punished" by powerful women. There is no anger or resentment. There is no whisper of shame about these fantasies of submission to a woman. But then, they are confiding to a very sympathetic ear.

I only became aware of women's sexual assertiveness in the workplace when I started working for a hospital. In this environment, women outnumber men, and they liked to embarrass me about my sexual performance. Once, a woman plopped a picture of a naked man with a huge schlong entertaining a fully clothed woman on top of my workstation. One of the female employees was an ardent feminist who didn't like men. I think she enjoyed giving orders to men and trying to intimidate them. At one of the first meetings I attended, she took her shoes off and started rubbing my leg under my pants. I tried to ignore it, not only because I was married, but because I knew in the long run, it would mess with my job.

Boy, did I jerk off to that one. I'd fantasize that I'm asked to attend a meeting at work, the only man there in the department. After listening for two hours, my powerhouse female boss says, "We are going to do something different now." She turns to me, "Have you ever heard of the concept of clothed females and nude males?"

"Yes," I say.

"Well, the females are all clothed. Why aren't you nude?"

"Well," I stammer.

"Off with the clothes."

She says she wants my clothes off because, as her employee, I'm to give an honest evaluation of her work and the work of all her female coworkers. She wants the naked truth of how I worship them. If my worship is convincing, I will be allowed to orally satisfy my superiors. I grovel at each of their feet, praising them until they reveal their vaginas. With my tongue, I'm allowed to bring them to climax.

I have a similar fantasy with my wife where she has a women's meeting and I end up the lone naked "guest."

Warren

In fantasies, we see men circle women, one minute dominating them, the next being dominated by them. Warren, a solder in the army and a confirmed romantic, speaks of fear of women's power in reality. He believes this may be the result of growing up with a dominating mother who was anti-sex. In fantasy, he is able to let go.

In a way, I am a little frightened as to the intensity of the major fantasy I have designed for my girlfriend, as it is so different from my lifelong idealized views on life and love. I thought I was mad, the only man in the world who really loved to be controlled by a woman. I started to fantasize from childhood. From the very beginning, I really loved to be controlled or be a slave of a beautiful woman. She makes me do whatever she likes. When I was fourteen, I got a chance to see a video of a "blue" film. One man was lying on a bed. A woman sat on his face, and another sat over his penis. He was licking her cunt so fast, and the other woman was pumping very fast. This scene changed my whole life. It was the day I learned to masturbate. I ran to my room and imagined that a girl I liked was sitting on my mouth and her girlfriend on my penis. She ordered me to suck her cunt and chew her clit like a chocolate. Unknowingly, my hands reached over to my penis, and I started to shake it very slowly. Oh, what a great experience it was! Within a few minutes, my juices reached the top of the ceiling, about fifty grams of thick, hot ice cream. From that day, I started to masturbate daily, five or six times, sometimes eight or nine times. My record, believe it or not, was twelve times within five hours. The eleventh and twelfth times I had pain, rather than pleasure, and instead of juice, there was a little water and air. I used to fuck and lick so many beautiful women in my dreams almost daily. But in real life, I never got one woman then.

What will we take from our experiences and what will we discard? Sometimes, seemingly inconsequential moments incorporate themselves into unforeseen aspects of our lives, manifesting sexual desires, fantasies that become a part of our makeup. For Spike, it's the beautiful teacher responsible for overlooking the boys' urination during their restroom breaks that becomes ever present, the authority figure, the dominant mother whom he needs to please, admire, be under the control of.

Spike

I am a divorced man with a graduate degree. My wife didn't like sex—a few people out there don't. She wasn't orgasmic, and as you can imagine, problems developed. I've been told that I'm a very sensitive lover; a couple of ladies have even said I'm their best ever. But no matter how hard I tried to help my wife enjoy sex, she never did. And I just love women and making love.

I realize many of our likes and dislikes arise from our early life and our surroundings. My mother, for example, was large-breasted, and I really like and appreciate large-breasted women. Because of my early experiences at school, I have a subconscious desire to pee in front of a lady, now that I am old enough to understand how sexy this could be for the right person. This could take place with her standing behind or to the side of me, maybe even holding my penis, and directing the flow. Ideally, it would end with her jacking me off or us sharing some great sex.

I think this desire harks back to a routine that existed in our elementary school. Today, looking back, it seems somewhat erotic. The principal of the school, an older, never-married lady, had a rule that all teachers must accompany us during our three-times-a-day restroom breaks. All the teachers were female, and, as I remember, my third-grade teacher was quite young and pretty. She had full view of our private parts, which, even if someone wanted to be modest and shield her from view, couldn't without peeing on his neighbor. Penises have a mind of their own, too. No one ever got aroused in her presence; it was just like having your mom standing there, I guess. No one ever masturbated in front of her. Even as young as fifth or sixth grade, I remember some of the boys had pretty good-sized penises, which I didn't. Also, many young boys while peeing don't hold their penises because they just naturally stick out at a forty-five degree angle and don't point toward one's feet, as they seem to do as men age. Once in a while, her face would become pink, which was no doubt a blush.

I related this to a story a lady friend told me a few years back. One of her girlfriends had a baby boy whose penis was extremely large, extending just short of his knee. When it was time to change his diapers, all of her female friends would be sure to accompany her so they could *see it. Some would even make comments such as, "I'd like to know him when he's eighteen," etc. I realized then that many ladies do enjoy looking, as our teachers probably did, too.*

I wondered how/if the images of these women admiring the baby boy's penis will affect his future, his fantasies. Will he crave the admiration of his penis or gain pleasure in withholding it?

Jesse, a young man in his early thirties, raised by his full-figured mother and aunts, remembers massaging their sore feet to much appreciation. He now manifests his fantasy into a reality through online ads he posts, such as this (SSBBW = Super-Size Big Beautiful Woman):

Seeking SSBBW w/Extremely Thick FLAT Bare Feet

White male, 40, athletic seeks very heavy and obese women (300–400+ lbs) who would be into having their feet completely worshipped in every way. I am extremely infatuated with very heavy women and get kind of hypnotized by very thick, fleshy, flat-soled feet along with any other "imperfections" such as bunions, rough calloused skin, yellowed unkempt toenails, hammertoes, etc. I seek mature women over 40 who are serious about meeting. If you for any reason feel that this is too freaky or feel compelled to write negative opinions about what turns me on, please refrain. I am serious, honest, and for real

> *about what I am into so please only write and
> respond if you are mutually interested in being
> treated like a foot goddess where I worship your
> feet intensely and adoringly. Please do NOT
> respond if you are looking to email for weeks/
> months etc. I am trying to find someone who
> (like me) doesn't play games and wants to really
> meet ASAP.*

I am glad to be a woman, now more than ever. That the lesbian and gay worlds have grown to such acceptance has also seemed to me a part of this gender awakening. But I've always felt that women had greater potential for mental cruelty than men, perhaps a balance for having less muscle. When I was growing up, we girls knew how to twist the screws when one of us got more than her share. It was the meanest kind of pain, more wounding than a physical blow, especially when administered by one's "sister." Females are particularly good at the slow sadistic undoing of a person's sense of self, leaving the victim off-balance as to who they are, a far worse nightmare than physical torture. In our heart of hearts, most of us know that women are the scary ones. Put a woman who's a crazed killer in a movie and strong men shiver.

I remember when feminism was flowering and women's groups were forming all over Manhattan. The group to which I belonged was called "Women's Ink," and we numbered about thirty-five to forty women writers. We'd meet once a month in a member's apartment. We lasted less than six months. What blew us apart was "a whispering campaign" against a particular woman who happened to be bright, assertive, and, yes, very pretty. One of the founders of Women's Ink just couldn't abide this lovely woman's success at everything.

A couple of years later, I was in Los Angeles for a feminism powwow, maybe eight or nine of us. On our second night, we went bar-hopping in downtown LA, a part of town with which I was totally unfamiliar. We went to a club and when I turned around, the other three women were gone. Don't get me wrong, I was an adult and able to take care of myself, but this was supposed to be "the sisterhood," and I knew that getting rid of me wasn't by chance. They didn't like what I'd been saying at meetings. "Friday likes men too much" summed it up. I found a cab. I got back to the hotel, but I was deeply hurt inside as only I could be when other women are cruel to their own gender.

The next morning, I awoke with a burning anus. I hadn't a clue what it was. Scared and somewhat shamefaced, I called a nice older woman I'd met in LA. She told me to sit in a warm bath and get some Preparation H. I'm smiling as I write this, but I wasn't smiling then. That is how deeply abandonment by women affects us women. It went way back in time, that desertion by my feminist sisters, to being the third wheel of my mother and sister.

I tell the above stories not to demonize women but to include us in the human race. We are no better or worse than men. Men may be more proficient at physical abuse, but perhaps we step up with our adeptness at mental cruelty.

Domination, authority, throw in subjugation and control—all are strong words that interrupt our flow of thought and make us pay attention. Consider our fascination with each new murder, brutality, or rape as we watch TV. What does domination ignite? The answer, of course, is that state none of us can avoid: total dependency and domination by the first and foremost person "entitled" to control us. Today, we live in a time when mothers are no longer seen as "sanctified." Getting women off the throne of the all-good, all-benevolent Madonna frees up reality.

Has stripping mothers of their benevolence allowed us to see the source of women's capacity for domination and control? Certainly, women's swift adaptation into what was once a man's world says straightaway how adept women are at running things, being "on top."

Why was there panic in the '50s leading to arrests of men who solicited the suggestive dominatrix photos of Bettie Page? What was the threat? Men have always enjoyed the fantasy or fact of a woman taking them over, forcing them into submission, gagging them, tying them up, but this was a secret we were not meant to find out.

I predicted in *My Secret Garden* in the early '70s that "as women move more strongly into their recently won sexual freedom, and leave their historic role of second sex behind…they will, ironically, get into domination fantasies more and more. But the move will be in two directions. First, the new reality of being man's equal makes them unconsciously nervous about their identity as women, and so throws them back into longing for the traditional…dominating man; but second, they will want to explore and signal, even to themselves, their new liberated age by putting themselves into the dominant position of the sexual brute. Whether as brute or brutalized, in fantasy at least, the centuries of female submission are being avenged."

Now, in fantasy, women dream of the look and texture of a man's body. We are more into capturing the man, having him, owning him in ways unavailable to women in the past. Men are wary of women today and rightly so; we were always far more powerful and dominant in his eyes than in our own. Now we are here, strutting in and out of stilettos, breasts hoisted high as possible, and wallets as fat as his.

Who needs a whip?!

In an interview recently, a man told me, "I look forward to a female-dominated world." I responded, "It may not be much of a wait." The following Craigslist ads show that for those who want it, it's already here.

A DOM Asian woman searching her sub man – 37

A good looking, very fit, tall, single Asian woman seeking her sub Boy friend, love for a Long-term relationship. I am a normal person, little bit dominant side for mental controlling, spoiling. Not into pain, hardcore things, only looking for a submissive man here, not for Dominant man. pic to pic

In need of a alpha submissive

Submissive: A strong man, intelligent, driven, confident and passionate who leads all day. In his free time he seeks the comfort and freedom afforded by gifting his submission to a Dominant woman. He desires to lose control, wants to please in all ways, to become free through his submission.

Any Dominant women out there for LTR ???? — 49

This has been a monumental task, finding a truly Dominant woman who also wants a long term relationship with a wonderful attractive divorced white male who is looking to adore, worship & obey her.

This is not a sex game with me. I've had this type of relationship before and found it very fulfilling.

I simply cannot be happy in a plain old "vanilla" relationship.

I need a woman who enjoys being in charge, and having me be submissive to her in all ways, while infusing this is a relationship which will appear as a normal loving relationship in public and to family and friends, yet we know who I belong to in private. I am 5´11, 200, successful in shape, very attractive and sexy.

You should be over 32, slender or medium build, nice legs (for me to adore), disease free, open-minded, and have an idea how a Dom/ sub relationship should work.

This is very real and not a game.

Only those truly interested should inquire. We can discuss things more deeply when we speak by phone, as voice verification is required.

FANTASIES OF THE STRANGER
"Take Me, Whoever You Are!"

The Internet provides a New World enabling us to easily act out fantasies or just discover how common our fantasies are—fantasies we thought were reserved for us alone. Perusing the Craigslist ads, it's fascinating to see the similarities and differences between the sexes. Straight women may advertise for more romance, walking on the beach with that someone special. Lesbians tend to be more sexually adventurous, exploring something taboo. Straight men may also advertise for finding that special someone, although the underlying theme may have more sexual undertones, whereas gay men are the most sexually explicit. Ads such as the next one are not uncommon.

Italian BOTTOM needs raw pounding from TOP cock – 37

Looking to take on a big hot pole today, get you rock hard, then feel you pound my meaty butt like a bitch in heat. Masc 37 bottom, 5´10˝, 200 Italian br/br, 7˝c thick here with an incredibly sweet and juicy bubble butt. Pic below is my ass around a buddy's big thick tool. Please respond with a pic...not into surprises. Uninhibited and anon guys are cool.

For several years, Mitch has been posting: "Pound My Sweet Hole Raw! I'll be blindfolded, face down in bed, ass lubed, door open, come in, plant your seed, and go." Before the Internet, he only occasionally fulfilled this common dangerous fantasy of anonymity by visiting certain sex clubs. Since going online, it has been hard for him to not post this ad whenever time allows, even though he is knowingly putting his life in danger.

It's the rare family where children are raised to admire their genitals, enjoy masturbation, and anticipate sexual intercourse as an activity as enjoyable, acceptable, and responsible as driving the car. The fantasy of being taken by the faceless stranger allows us to enjoy guiltless sex with no emotional repercussions.

Bree

I'm a single mother raising my daughter while going to college to become a teacher. I had a difficult childhood. My mother was not there for me, mentally or physically. I was put in foster homes or stayed with friends of my mother's. I was molested from the age of six until I was thirteen. All of my molestations were men. I resent my mother for not being there to protect me. My father has never been a part of my life. He could not handle being a father. I have such disgust for him. But at the same time, I feel so sorry for him.

Boy, was I sexually active as a teenager. I did it with anybody who would screw me. I never used protection. All I did was tell the guy to pull out before he came. All that resulted in five pregnancies and four abortions. I don't like to masturbate at all. If a guy does it to me, I love it. But I am older now and much more careful, and I am damned lucky I'm still alive.

I fantasize a lot about men. I dream about men. I think about men all day. I am into X-rated books. I get real turned on by seeing a black guy getting it on with a white woman or two guys getting it on with a woman.

My favorite fantasy is that I am housekeeping when a man comes in the house and throws me against a wall and blindfolds me. I am so scared, but at the same time, I want this stranger to fuck me. This man is rubbing against me with his dick. I am moaning for him to put his finger into me, and he does, faster and faster. I tell him I want his dick in my cunt. He tells me to turn around, and he lays me down on the table and tells me I better be a good girl or he won't give me a good fuck. But first he tells me to go down on him. I tell him I have never done this before. He gets mad and gets on top of me and rams his dick into my throbbing cunt, his balls flapping against my body. I cum in spasms.

Sherry

Finding sexual pleasure is a large gift, and it was even more so for me. I'm almost thirty-three years old, married for seven years to a man I adore, and I have been with him for almost eleven years. My sexual history is simple from one point of view—I've never had sex with anyone other than my husband—and complex from another. After having intercourse with him for about nine months, I developed a condition called vaginismus. My vagina muscle closed involuntarily when anything tried to penetrate it. I also went through phases where I didn't want my husband to touch me sexually.

I had this condition for about six years before I discovered it was a problem shared by other people and found professional help. It took three years with a really great therapist and a very patient and understanding husband to work my way to wanting and being able to have intercourse. I thought my family history was normal, but it was actually one of neglect and intense emotional isolation. This led to problems I had never identified in trusting, communicating, and connecting with others, including my husband, and these problems all became focused in my vagina. Finding ways to turn my body on and achieve orgasm using tools such as fantasy was crucial to my wanting intercourse again.

In my favorite fantasy, it is summer, and I am in a crowded subway station waiting for a train. It's hot and sticky, even with the air conditioning. I'm a bit sweaty. I'm small-breasted, so I can get by without a bra, and it's too hot for panties. When the subway doors open, I am swept on in a gigantic flood of people. When the doors close, I find myself pressed up against a metal pole, hemmed in by a wall of humanity. The heat from all those bodies against and around me is intense. As I cling to the pole for dear life, I become aware of a body behind me, a masculine body, pressing into my back. There is nowhere to even shift my weight given the press of people around me. Then, I feel his penis through the back of my thin skirt, hardening and rubbing. It feels gentle, questioning, and urgent.

I lean slightly back into him to show my interest. I lift up my shirt to feel the cold metal against my breasts. I rub my clit up and down the pole. I can feel myself groaning although it is drowned out by the noise of the train. He's got his penis lengthwise against my skirt. He knows he is driving me crazy. That's his purpose. His hands move up under my skirt to caress my hips and buttocks. My juices run helplessly with sweat pouring down my legs. He's hiked my skirt so high that my clitoris is bare against the pole now. Then, the loudspeaker announces the next stop, and the train starts to slow. Finally his cock starts, teasing for a moment, just a bit, in and out, so I am sure I will die right there on the spot. The ripples inside me get longer and more intense until they explode in a series of spasms that feel like they're moving the pole along with me to the other end of the train. As the last one dies and I cling limply to the pole, the doors of the train open, and he is gone with the rush of exiting commuters.

FANTASIES OF SPANKING
"So, That's What a Brush Is For!"

I look at the women I know, bright, brilliant, beautiful, some of them leaders in their field, and yet, still today, most would be offended if you called them dominating.

We women used to pretend that the ability to discipline was not in us. We were the softer, gentler sex. While women raised the human race—the most formidable job on Earth—we were only "girls, ladies," dependent on men who ran the show. Those few exceptions were considered almost depraved, certainly not a real woman. There was nothing more unladylike you could say about a woman than to accuse her of being "dominating, domineering."

Men took on the role of "the heavy." They were assigned "punishment duty," as in "Wait till your father gets home!" At the same time, children in their hearts knew that no one really had more influence over them than the woman who bore and raised them. It was often confusing to accept that the tired man who came home at the end of the day was The Enforcer. Nonetheless, movies and television backed up this division of roles within the family—with sweet sitcom shows like *Father Knows Best* and *Leave It to Beaver*.

Thank God, women no longer look stunned when you tell them to stop being so bossy. The jaw may drop, a plaintive protest on the tip of their tongue, but then reality strikes. The woman shrugs, owns up to that side of herself with which she's still not comfortable, and changes the subject.

With women out of the home now for several decades, has the lack of discipline in real life led to more discipline in fantasy? Children have grown up with a hunger for discipline, for someone in control. Many families no longer eat dinner together, each person grabbing something from the fridge, throwing it in the microwave, to suit their own schedule. By the time these children are in their twenties and thirties—such as many of the young men and women in this book—the taste for what was missing in childhood is fixed. Although fantasies of spanking are often traced back to the discipline of the commander in chief of the home, the all-powerful caretaker's hand, it is not exclusively the case. Control, and losing it, are often what sex is all about.

Luis

I'm a twenty-nine-year-old single man. Both my parents worked and were pretty lenient. I was never hit, rarely punished, the worst I was given was a stern talking to. I probably would've misbehaved more if I thought it would've led to a good spanking instead of a boring lecture. My spanking fantasies went back to when I was very young. I used to read lots of superhero comic books when I was a kid, and I remember there was one issue of Superboy *where Lana Lang was pictured over her father's knee about to take a spanking with a hairbrush. I found if I laid on the floor and moved my groin up and down when I looked at that picture, I used to get a very nice feeling indeed. Still today, nothing gets me as excited as thinking about a strong woman taking a paddle to my butt.*

Barry

Barry, a young man from Britain, is in his longest relationship. He was never physically disciplined by his parents but remembers very vividly being spanked over the teacher's knee along with several of his boyhood classmates in grade school.

When I was about twenty-six, I was working up in London, and I was not seeing anyone. There used to be lots of cards in phone boxes for "Strict Mistresses" or "Naughty Schoolgirls," and one day, I couldn't resist. I phoned and arranged to see one of these prostitutes. She was an exceptionally pretty girl of the type I have always liked. I felt very embarrassed telling her that I wanted her to cane me, but she took it all in her stride as if it were perfectly normal. She gave me the cane and then the whip on my bare bottom and then asked if I wanted anything else. I paid fifty pounds for sexual intercourse. "How do you like it?" she asked. "Could you go on top?" I answered, and she smiled very sexily.

Sally

I'm twenty-two, black, and graduated from a major East Coast liberal arts college. I work for a well-known magazine and am trying to publish a book of poetry. I'm very open-minded about people's sexuality and fetishes, and I expect people to feel the same about me. I took a human sexuality class and a sociology and sexual diversity class that helped me come to grips with my own sexuality and that of others. It has helped me find a peace of mind that I couldn't accomplish in therapy.

In my fantasy, I imagine myself as a lusty and insatiable woman who has to be reprimanded by her man. (Usually, he is a faceless man, but once in a while, he's my boyfriend.) I have an hourglass figure, huge, buoyant, perky breasts that want to pop out of my tiny black bra. My nipples are big and rosy. I traipse around the house wearing a sheer blouse and a short flared skirt. Underneath, I am wearing thigh-high stockings and a thong bikini. On my feet, I am wearing three-inch heels. My lover comes in and is angry because I've disobeyed him and worn these trashy clothes. He is very angry. He pushes me over the table and pulls down my panties. He gives me twenty hard spanks with a hairbrush, and he sees my clit growing in ecstasy. He spanks me harder and harder until my ass is swollen.

He tells me he is going to give me what I've been craving. He spreads whipped cream all over my sore ass until it is slippery and shiny. He then stuffs his dick into my puckering asshole. (I really don't like anal sex in real life.) He shoves it in and out, and we are both moaning like idiots. He pulls out and shoves it in my pussy. We are doing it doggy style. I can feel his balls hitting my clitoris, and I am absolutely insane. We both cum screaming frantically. In real life, I am pretty orgasmic at this point and hope that my boyfriend smells my turned-on pussy and shoves his tongue or dick into it. (In reality, it is very hard for me to have an orgasm, but I'm not sure why.)

In fantasies of domination, we abdicate responsibility. In the olden days, women weren't raised to be responsible for sex; yes, we were responsible for *not* having sex—until marriage—but we weren't raised to initiate sex, to even think we were sexual creatures, but instead were made to believe that until a man "turned us on," like a light switch, we were devoid of sex. This belief was possible to accept, since we weren't allowed to even masturbate, the most logical exercise in the world for teaching sexual responsibility and know-how.

Prior to adolescence, I was eager to initiate almost anything. But came Cinderella time, the captain of the team, the leader of the girl pack, I took smaller steps and learned to wait to be asked, to practice assiduously the "virtue" of passivity. It was hard. In those bygone days, it was maddening to wait, for those of us who were naturally inclined to telephone the boy, ask him to dance.

Adolescents today are forging new territory. Girls raised by women who have mother-power and economic power don't take no for an answer. Today, many young girls do just this; they walk up, hold out their hand, shrug if they are rejected, and try the next guy or girl.

FANTASIES OF RAPE
"Stop! No! Please! Stop!...Why'd You Stop?"

Young girls are formidable creatures. Even in the old days, adolescent boys had their work cut out for them, given female drive and determination. Today, young women's fantasies are often full of vindictive anger at men for what they see online, in movies, on television as well as what they hear from their mothers, not to mention what they experience in real life. Today's young women often retaliate, imagining themselves in fantasy as the dominatrix; is it seduction or rape that excites them? Whether bondage, pain, or punishment, these women's orgasms are often laced with revenge.

Why is the rape fantasy today still so prevalent, even for those who have never been raped nor desire it? Does it go back to a time not long ago when women were not allowed to be sexual? Even today, do many women think of the kind of "pow-erful/rough" sex that they want as inappropriate for them? In fantasies of rape, their desires are not in question; it is beyond their control.

For actual victims of rape, such as Melly, the fantasies can also be very therapeutic.

Melly

Let me comfort my boyfriend and all men by saying that monogamy is more sensual than anything that goes on in my head. I love my boyfriend and would never trade what we have for any of my mental affairs that may have a chance of becoming reality. My fantasies are usually about rape or lesbianism. Both I have experienced—only the latter would I enjoy again. The lesbian fantasies are always "soft and plush," whereas the rape fantasies are cruel and hard. Sometimes, I have a reverse rape fantasy in which the man who really did rape me is on his back, crying for more. I say, "How do you like it, mutha fuckah?" I feel so relieved after I cum, sometimes the happiness makes me cry. I suggest fantasy for any woman who has been raped.

Nicole

I'm twenty-three now, but when I was in high school, my parents wouldn't let me date. When I graduated high school, I started going to bars as soon as I could get into them. I always carried condoms with me. But I began to feel I should control my life and not just let things happen. Most men my age seem so immature and irresponsible.

I have become interested in female domination porn, which I don't think is degrading to women. The women are mostly clothed and the men nude. Since I don't like to look at women, this is perfect. I also like the feeling of power I get from seeing men submissive to women. The men seem eager to please women, unlike the traditional porn most men look at. I've never tried anything I've seen on anyone I've met but have fantasized about it. I've chatted online with a few subjects but haven't had the nerve to meet. I am particularly aroused by the scenes of women raping men.

I have a rape fantasy, where in a funny way, I'm in control. I am in bondage. I tell them the rules that they can play by. One is no ejaculating on me; they must all wear condoms. While each one fucks me, the others must watch. I ask them all to tell me exactly how each feels about women, to let loose verbally with all the anger they've ever felt. I ask them to tie me to the bed. The first man gets on top of me. He says, "You're a whore, a dirty bitch." The anger in his voice is intense. I can see the expressions on the other men's faces, and they all display desire. All the others can't wait their turns. You see, I choose the next guy I want to fuck.

I believe strongly in guilt-free imagined fantasies wherein we are in total control and no one gets hurt. In women's relatively new role as men's equal, it is one thing to feel at home with power during the day at work, but when the day is done and our clothes are off, our breasts bare, nipples hard, and our vagina moist, and that pulsating sensation within crying for someone's mouth or the entry of a stiff cock, we often don't want to lead or instruct. *We want to be taken!* Many of these women say up front that they "hate real domination," but in fantasy, it makes them wet, makes them fly out of this tense difficult world.

What relieves our responsibility for sexual satisfaction more than being forcibly taken by one man or woman and also feeds into our exhibitionistic and voyeuristic sides? Answer: being taken by many men and women.

FANTASIES OF GROUP FORCE
"When One Man Is Too Much and a Hundred Are Too Many"

Sarah

Sarah, who is thirty-three and well-educated, has opted out of or "not followed up," her words, in many sexual situations, leaving them to remain only sexual fantasies. She admits, in real life, the man who is the basis of the following fantasy was probably given mixed signals.

I have many different fantasies—which usually include two men—and sometimes women. To me, having sex with two people at the same time feeds my psychological need for more. My parenting wasn't enough.

Part of this fantasy actually happened when I was away from home on a two-month job. After sitting in a dining room having breakfast and trying to look self-assured because I'm the only woman in the room, I was followed discreetly by a forty-year-old man in a suit and tie. He ended up asking me to come to his room. I told him, "No." But later, when I left work, a car pulled up alongside me, and the same man asked if I would reconsider the offer.

This is where the fantasy starts. I say it will cost him. He then says if he's paying, he wants me to dress like a schoolgirl. So, later, I knock on his hotel door, dressed as a schoolgirl. He says I can come in as long as I don't mind his friend being there. The first man sits me on his lap, and at this point, the second man squats down on the floor and peels back my shirt. They then take off my skirt. Still with my panties on, the first man slides his hand down and slips a big finger into my tight, fresh hole. He begins working it in and out slightly. The second man comments that all my juices are dribbling everywhere, and with that, he pulls my panties down to my ankle and started to lick at the juices and then deeper toward my cunt.

Lucas

A forest ranger in the northern Midwest, Luke is married to a teacher. They have two children and find they have less and less time to spend together and less energy for sex than they used to.

I should say that I was never able to play the macho role very well. I got into forestry not because I was some kind of lumberjack or Boy Scout type, but because I became very interested in the environmental movement in college and developed an interest in environmental science.

A few years ago, my wife and I started to tell each other fantasy stories as we made love. This verbal fantasizing helped make sex a lot more fun for both of us. My problem is that I want to act out more of these fantasies, and she does not. I can occasionally persuade her to dress up in sexy corsets, black stockings, boots, etc. She has been willing to tie me up a couple of times. But I usually have to ask her to do these things; she does not do them on her own initiative. However, I don't really enjoy acting out as much as I do the fantasies. We don't really play the parts well. It's better for me to fantasize about these things and for us to tell each other our fantasies.

In my fantasy, I am driving a very expensive sports car through the mountains of California. I am taking curves real fast and loving every minute of it. I look in my rearview mirror and notice that a motorcycle cop is following me. I decide to try to outrun the cop but "he" keeps following me. Finally, on a dangerous curve, I lose control of the car and spin around. The cop manages to avoid crashing into me, stops the motorcycle, and starts walking toward me.

I look up and see the gun pointed at me. I hear, "Out of the car, asshole." I realize that the cop is a woman. She is a lot stronger and quicker than I am. She turns around so that she's facing me. She says, "You're under arrest for reckless driving. If you try anything, you'll wish you hadn't." She tells me to get on her motorcycle, behind her. She starts up quickly. She enjoys taking risks when she drives. After a fast drive up some mountain roads, we stop at a remote chalet. "Get off," she says. My hands are handcuffed behind me. She takes out her gun and motions me toward the house. "Inside," she says.

We walk inside a beautiful chalet. There is a cathedral ceiling, several pillars, a sunken living room, and a large stone fireplace with a roaring fire. The carpet is white. She quickly unlocks my handcuffs and then handcuffs me again behind a pillar. She ties my legs together. She sits down on a large, soft white couch. She is still dressed in her police uniform, leather jacket, boots, etc.

"What are you going to do with me?" I ask.

"Don't be a pussy," she says.

A man walks in. He is six-foot-five and very well-built. She looks at me, and I know I am to say nothing. The man acts as if I'm not there. Suddenly, she springs up and tackles him. She is stronger than he is. She wrestles him and then handcuffs him to another pillar. She unzips both of our pants and takes our cocks out. She realizes we are both helpless and laughs. "Let's play a game," she says. She picks up her nightstick and holds it down by her cunt. "I'll suck the first one whose cock gets as big as this. The other one has to watch." She starts to masturbate. We can't do anything about our own cocks, but we know what they want to do.

A woman comes in. She is dressed in running clothes and is out of breath. She is the wife of the other man. "We're seeing who has the biggest cock," the cop says. The other woman takes off her clothes. They go over to the couch and start doing 69 on each other. This makes the two of us even hornier. Finally, they cum, both at the same time.

The cop goes over to the other man and pours a drink over his cock, then starts licking him. He cums very quickly. She then walks over to me. She licks the semen off her lips as she does this. "What do you want?" she says.

"I want to fuck you," I say.

"Beg."

She pushes me down on my knees, turns to the other woman, and says, "What do you think?"

"I'll fuck him," the other woman says.

She unlocks my handcuffs and motions me toward the other woman. I start to walk toward her, but she trips me, and I fall on the floor. She jumps on top of me, turns me over, and fucks me quickly.

We see the male population today divided with regard to the joy of women's sexual emancipation. There are men who fantasize about women becoming madly orgasmic and wildly out of control sexually, while others hold on to male domination, with women available for man's sexual pleasure. Is the latter a defense against full awareness of the total power a woman once held over him—the power, if he is not careful, that could easily be relinquished again? Or is it to deny the hunger some women have for sex? A cuckolded man—should she look elsewhere or succumb to the mailman—in some men's eyes is no man at all.

I can understand why a male-dominated society puts blinders and boundaries on women's sexuality. Patriarchal men so feared the depth and energy of women's sexuality, they deprived themselves of sexually responsive wives. It was the only way they could leave home for work and not wonder what the little woman was up to. I recently came across the following online site.

Married Women Dating Community!

Have you ever dated a married woman? Well this is your chance to check out this 'Lonely Wives Dating' network, and you can do it for NO COST at all. Come on, you have to admit that you're a little curious.

Listening to the fantasies of women as well as their actual sexual adventures, I understand why men went to such lengths not to be cuckolded. Augusta, a middle-aged married woman, says, "My fantasies usually do center around some type of domination trip, which is odd, since I detest the thought of being dominated by anyone, male or female, in real life and have had real adjustment problems because of this issue." She goes on to emphasize, "Some male researchers have commented that women's sex desire is small. *Absolutely not true.* Sometimes, my feelings are so intense that they really get in the way of my daily routine."

Men would never have so rigidly insisted on their right to patriarchy and control—stripping women of all sexual initiative, depriving themselves of great sex at home—if they hadn't been aware of the power of women when they were growing up. Though the world is shifting on its axes and women have joined the ranks of fans of the domination fantasy, it is still primarily the fantasy playground of men.

Tucker

Tucker is a middle-aged man married for thirty-seven years to a woman he describes as "the most wonderful woman in the world." He, like Ian earlier in this chapter, has the typical man-on-top fantasy. Does letting go, losing control, submitting, reawaken fears of being controlled by a dominant mother?

In our relationship, I have always been the dominant one and Mary the passive/submissive one. We both like it very much this way. There is no pain to our lovemaking, yet I always dominate her, and this pattern of dominance all began way back when I was in the third grade. I would pretend that I had a beautiful girl tied up naked to a tree, and I would beat her with a rope. I think this came from seeing my mother as the dominant force in our family and my father never standing up to her, but I'm not sure.

Anyway, one day, I mentioned my fantasies to my wife, Mary. When I am on top of her, fucking her, I fantasize:

One, she is my sex slave and being forced to submit to my pleasures.

Two, as I fuck her, there are several men standing around us urging me to fuck her harder and faster.

Three, I am only one of several men who are gang-raping her. I am the fourth or fifth to fuck her, and there are others waiting in line.

Four, I am a soldier, and the other soldiers and I have captured her, and she must do everything we tell her—anal, oral, and coital to each of us.

Mary enjoys acting out her role as a sex slave during our time of foreplay, which can and has lasted for a couple of hours or more before we even get into oral, anal, or coital. For instance, she will go into the bedroom and put on whichever outfit I order her to wear; i.e., she will come into the living room wearing a knee-length skirt, hose, heels, garter belt, no panties, a sleeveless low-cut blouse, and no bra. She will stand in front of me and say, "Is this what you want, master?"

I will say, "Yes," and order her to spread her legs, lift her dress to her waist, and she will obey immediately, letting me get a vision of the prettiest and cleanest shaved pussy any woman would hope to have.

I, like many women, have always chafed under the rules of patriarchy. Even with the kindest husband, some wives feel the power balance within the relationship as controlling. Until we are married, women know that our lives belong to us and are ours to invest. Growing up, we may have had strict parents, but there were ways of avoiding their control over us.

Losing interest in sex after marriage has a great deal to do with the feeling of having lost one's independence. Under patriarchy, women ran the home, raised the children, but total dependence on a husband for the bread on the table and the roof over their heads smothered that spark that ignites eros.

Many of the women who write about their domination fanta-sies have been abused at some point in their lives. Tessa says, "I grew up with a father who was an alcoholic. He was a senior po-lice officer and violent in every way possible to me. Over the last eight years, a lot of my fantasies have revolved around domina-tion and being at the mercy of an older, controlling, brutal man."

It's fascinating having lived in both worlds, pre- and post-feminism. If I evoke the pre-feminist world so often, it's to make sense out of our fantasies as well as our real lives in a world that is changing at an unprecedented rate. To understand our sexual behavior nowadays—not just what we do but how we feel about ourselves sexually—it helps to remember three levels of change. The quickest thing to change is our attitude about sex. It can be triggered by nothing more than the relaying of a friend's experience.

What changes more slowly is our sexual behavior. Nina, a "single, white, college-educated virgin…technically," says, "As a child and adolescent, my fantasies were mostly based on being seduced/dominated by men. However, as an adult, my fantasies have made a complete change, in that now I am usually the one dominating the man. Depending on my mood, my fantasies will range from playful to cruel."

Third level, the slowest to change—if it changes at all within our lifetime—are our deepest, often unconscious feelings about our bodies and our sexual behavior, attitudes we learned from our parents.

We seek to be free of the burden of these feelings by turning over control. Or finally controlling them through domination now that feminism has laid the groundwork for young girls to carry leadership skills straight into adolescence.

Zoe

I consider myself to be a good-looking, assertive, heterosexual recovering alcoholic. I lost my virginity at nineteen but was masturbating by the age of ten. The first experience with masturbation that I can recall was with a bar of soap. That was replaced by running water, which continued for many years. Erotica has always been very stimulating—I love romance novels but look for the "explicit sex" disclaimers on the cover. I am quite adept at losing myself in a book. When I meet a man who is attractive, I usually fantasize a lot about him; that he desires me, can't resist me, thinks about me all the time. It's because, even though I'm told I'm good looking, subconsciously I still have to convince myself of it. I'm not strong on sexual confidence in reality, but I'm a powerhouse in my dreams. I would love to be pursued by an attractive man and tell him, "No!" all the time. It's old-fashioned but a real turn-on for me.

When it gets down to the nitty-gritty of really getting off, I think about bondage and being overwhelmed by a man. I imagine myself helpless, forced to be pleasured beyond human endurance by a watchful audience.

My favorite fantasy is being drugged and awakened to find strangers holding my legs spread wide open and my arms flung wide. There are several clothed men in the room with video cameras all focused on me. One gorgeous naked man approaches, reaches to spread my pussy wide so that I can be seen by all cameras, and he starts making tight circles on my clitoris with his finger. Another naked man comes over and holds my pussy lips wide apart. It all has a porno movie feel to it. I can see his cock dangling above my chest, pulsing. He starts delving his tongue into my vagina until I'm dying for release, but he pulls away before I can climax.

At this point, two beautiful women come to either side of me wearing nothing but open lab coats. They blindfold me and start sucking my

*nipples. I can feel their silky hair brushing along my ribs and stomach.
As I writhe and moan, they nibble my nipples, making soothing sounds.
Every time I come close to release, they suspend their activities. All
the while the two men are manipulating my vagina and clitoris. More
people come, and they are sucking my fingers and toes. I am sucking a
firm breast, and still they won't let me cum. I am lost in all their bodies,
and they are all making love to me.*

While many women now own their fantasies of domination,
some women seem puzzled by their fantasies of being dominated
because they are not like this "in real life." But isn't that the point?
Fantasies often counter, often try to get what we don't have in
reality. Men have always been into domination. It was thrust
upon them. Women have begun to learn what men have always
known—that while it's empowering to have authority, it can be
very tiring. To compensate for this sexually, more men and women
are getting into being "taken," being made to lie back and accept
the orgasm "beyond my control." It can be heard up and down the
halls of authority where we bring ourselves to erotic life with a
quick fantasy of being made, forced to let go the reins of power.

And when the day is finally over, and there's no one there to
cook dinner and take care of us, we have choices. To go out, go
online, search for a new love or just an exciting moment of satisfaction. Or we can run a warm bath, close our eyes, and pretend
in fantasy that the sensation mounting between our legs and
spreading to our brain, erasing all thoughts of responsibility, is
being aroused by our dream partner, that person in fantasy who
will not take no for an answer.

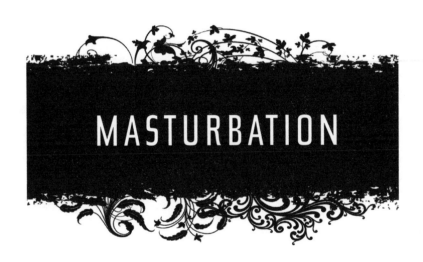

MASTURBATION

MASTURBATION

I feel it appropriate to say a few words in honor of masturbation when writing a new book about sex. A big word—masturbation—four syllables full of weight within the family where it is seldom mentioned, a silence that speaks with more force than words. "No, don't masturbate, my darling," was never said, though we are absolutely sure of mother's opinion.

Most of us are like thieves. We touch our bodies, all the while imagining mother's footsteps in the hallway, the dire consequence of her discovery, and our expulsion from the garden. In time, this imminent threat becomes fuel for the fire of our orgasm. Ah, the fantasy of almost getting caught! Getting away with our orgasm becomes part of who we are. Fact is, we want our mothers diametrically opposed to what we are doing when we put our hand between our legs; we want to keep mother dear asexual, while we ourselves are bad, bad, bad!

Long before boys entered my young life, there was nothing that raced my adrenaline like putting things that weren't mine into my pocket. Oh, the thrill at Woolworths, the rapid heartbeat as I walked away from the site of my crime! What if I'd been caught, and I, the president of my class, the straight-A student? I was a true Jekyll and Hyde, an identity I carried into adolescence when a boy's lips on mine spoke of the most forbidden fruit.

We're raised on stolen sex, beginning with masturbation. Early on, stealth becomes integral to our sexual history. Lying in bed at night, ears attuned to parental activity—are they up and about?—we bring ourselves to orgasm, the explosion thrilling at getting away with it. How could thievery of our own bodies not be a part of our ongoing sexual history? In time, we lie in a boy's arms in a parked car, the dark night all about us, and we feel his hand move between our legs. Our eyes closed, we give ourselves over to what we felt touching our bodies in our virginal bed, only now intensified a thousand times over.

We are creative artists, making stolen sex work for us in fantasy. Little did we know back then that, years later and miles away, the scary possibility of approaching footsteps would be the foundation and inspiration of our adult fantasy.

I once believed that the most salient difference between men's and women's fantasies was men's delight in imagining women bringing themselves to orgasm as opposed to women's total disinterest in men gratifying themselves. I still find it interesting that many men feel that "women don't want sex, really want it like men do." Perhaps men fantasize watching a woman masturbate in order to say, "Wow, she loves it as much as I do!"

I've known women to admit a certain jealousy or resentment of their man's fondness for masturbation. But I've never heard the reverse. It's not that women simply turned the idea over in their heads and rejected it. The subject never came up. For most women, a man bringing himself to orgasm was more of a turn-off than a turn-on, possibly because it made her feel unnecessary. Or was it her grudging certainty that a man is connected to his penis in a fond and intimate way that we women don't share with regard to our vagina? In any case, the penis didn't have the allure that the vagina had for straight men.

There were certainly exceptions to this rule, but it seemed to me that women who couldn't get enough of the penis—looking at it, watching it grow in our hands—tended to be fatherless girls who grew up in a home with no penis in residence. As women have now entered almost every exclusive "Boys' Club," perhaps we're also garnering their fantasies.

Someone once told me, "No one's going to make a thriving business out of peep shows for women that show guys masturbating." But the Internet has opened new doors. How many more women, raised by both parents, now visit sites devoted to male masturbation, sites that advertise to both men and women?

Over the years, more and more letters and emails, such as the one following by Susannah, show women raised by both parents increasingly turned on by male masturbation. We are no longer just the exhibitionists and males the voyeurs. More than ever, we are equals and can equally view men solely for our own pleasure as sexual objects. Perhaps there's a good reason why the term "boy toy" didn't appear until the late twentieth century.

THE BOY TOY HAS COME— HALLELUJAH!

Susannah

Susannah, from a conservative military family, has parents who never discussed sex. And any displays of nudity were looked on with embarrassment. In high school, with her first boyfriend, she discovered: "What a thrill it was to kiss, to have the boy touch my breasts, or to feel his erect penis through his clothes. The first time I felt that hard shaft against my stomach was wonderful because I knew I had done that to him." Like so many people from sexually repressed parents, she experienced the duality, outwardly the "proper" good girl with the secret "hot-blooded" sexually insatiable side. "One time, with a special boy, I managed twelve orgasms in two nights...okay, he was very special." After becoming pregnant, she married at age twenty.

Zach was a lousy lover, many sexual hang-ups, and after about eight years, I became attracted to Bob, a married coworker of Zach's. We began a correspondence that was initially innocent, and I discovered he was also attracted to me. This was the state of my sexual fantasies. *I used to fantasize about him every day and masturbate in the shower by letting the water pound my clitoris until I came. These fantasies were quite innocent in the beginning, kissing, etc. Later, as my confidence and my knowledge of reciprocated desire increased, I expanded my vision to include sex outdoors, on the dining room table, in front of the fireplace, etc. One was a particular favorite: Dressed only in a coat and high boots, I would go to Bob's office just before he was about to leave, lock the door, and seduce him. I would end up seated in his lap, impaled on his shaft, with the coat open and his face buried in my breasts. I was very frustrated in those days and actually had a couple of group sessions with my best friend's husband.*

This relationship didn't go anywhere. Then, after another couple of years, I rediscovered sexual fantasies when I was on the verge of becoming totally non-orgasmic again. This is the fantasy that allowed me to cum almost every single time we had sex during the last seven years of our marriage. It is early on a beautiful spring Sunday morning, and I have just come out of the shower. The weather is warm, so I take the newspaper and sit in a lounge chair on my apartment balcony, wearing just my long floral cotton bathrobe. By the way, I am no different from my real self in any way. As I am reading, a motion caches my eye, and I look over to the next apartment building in this cluster, where I find I can see into an apartment on the next lower floor. (In this fantasy,

I have terrific vision, which allows me to see all sorts of details that would normally be invisible at this distance.)

A man in his thirties, a good-looking stranger with curly light brown hair, is lying in bed, just under a sheet. The motion that caught my eye is his yawning and stretching as he wakes up. I see that he is quite handsome, with a tanned, moderately muscular body. After rubbing his hands over his face and through his hair, he glances down the sheet to the place where his morning erection has caused the sheet to lift, and he smiles to himself. Then, he flips the sheet away and lies there totally nude. Sun-bleached hair curls on his legs, arms, and lightly across his chest. His body is gorgeous, and I can't take my eyes off him. His average-sized penis, released from the sheet, stands almost straight up. He touches it lightly and grins as he watches it bounce. Reaching into a drawer in his night stand, he takes out something and does something to his hands. Although I cannot see clearly, it suddenly dawns on me that he must be rubbing lubricant on his hands in preparation for masturbation! I am full of anticipation, as I have never seen a man jerk off before.

Then, he wraps his hand around the shaft and begins to stroke it up and down slowly, almost lazily. After a few minutes of this, he releases the shaft, and I notice it is longer, thicker, and redder, although still of average size (no giant penises in my fantasies). My paper has dropped to the floor of the balcony, and I am feeling flushed. With one hand, he begins to play with his balls while the other hand reaches up to caress one of his nipples. I find that my right hand is creeping between my legs while the other begins to play with one of my nipples. The hair between my legs is moist with more than the water from the shower, and the labia are beginning to swell.

Now we are masturbating in tandem—as he pulls at his nipples and rolls them with his fingers, I do the same to mine, feeling the firm flesh on my breasts, too. He pumps his shaft and caresses his balls as lightly as I tease my clitoris and rub my mons. I have totally forgotten that I am outside in broad daylight, with my bathrobe wide open and my body displayed for all to see. Sometimes, he stops abruptly and just rubs his hands over his body and down his thighs while his penis bounces and quivers as though it were alive and begging for more. I do the same, stroking my body while my nipples ache with desire and my hips gyrate as my clitoris seeks any available stimulation in the absence of my fingers. Then, his hands resume their actions, and I am almost frenzied now as I rest myself, waiting for that magical moment when his penis will spasm and his hot fluid will shoot out. As I approach my orgasm, my body demands more sensation until I am squeezing and pinching my nipples and rubbing my clitoris firmly. Suddenly, his back arches, and he writhes, and both hands wrap around his shaft as white, hot cum shoots up and onto his chest. I plunge two fingers into my spasming vagina, clamping my other hand on top of them, writhing and gasping as I cum more violently. As I relax and my vision clears, I see the man lying back with a big smile of satisfaction and know that I have an identical smile on my face. (This, by the way, is exactly how I masturbate—except not where I can be seen!)

Sometimes, I add another part: As I lie there on the balcony, waiting for my breathing to slow down, I hear a gentle chuckle and look up to see on a balcony opposite and above mine—a strange man with dark hair and a moustache who has obviously been watching me! He is wearing only shorts or swim trunks, and his erection is quite visible. I find that I am only slightly embarrassed. This is where the fantasy ends. It worked every time unless I was coming down with something, so no wonder my husband thought he was the world's greatest lover.

OUR VAGINA IS DIRTY, SMELLY, NEVER TO BE MENTIONED, AND TO BE SAVED FOR THE MAN WE LOVE

What do we find so alluring about "the handsome stranger"? Our own sense of newness with a hero of unlimited fantasy, foreign hands tentatively cupping our breasts, spreading our legs, and a mouth, oh, my God, hot breath, lips, a tongue licking that part of us! For all our bravado, "it" remains open to judgment with each new love. Only in fantasy can we be absolutely sure that he loves the forbidden fruit he is eating.

In the popular fantasy of the stranger, "the hunk," is the desire for something more. He drifts into town and gets the women all hot and bothered. The play *Picnic* and the movie *Dirty Dancing* come to mind. We in the audience intuitively understand the ingénue's desire to reject the Nice Guy and risk everything with the Bad Boy, whose forbidden aura makes him absolutely appropriate for sex. Yet, we wonder why shy young girls, with their whole lives ahead of them, risk everything for a taste of forbidden sex. The answer is in front of us: if you have a "sewer" between your legs where no Nice Girl goes on her own, of course you hand it over to the Bad Boy, who yearns to go there, to bury his tongue, his lips.

Tammy

Tammy, who fantasizes making it with a stranger as she masturbates, writes that she has "dark hair, a curvy figure, and large breasts." When she was eighteen, a lot of men started asking her out. But she goes on to admit that because of a fear of getting hurt, now, at twenty-three, she's quite choosy and has only met a few men in her life that she's really sexually attracted to, an attraction that is as much mental as physical.

I have a recurring fantasy of asking this stranger to come with me for a cigarette, then leading him round the corner of the building where we can be alone. I am wearing a short skirt, knee-high boots, and no knickers. He immediately realizes what's on my mind and gives me a huge grin that tells me it's been on his mind too. We start kissing and gently run our hands all over each other's bodies. I want to feel his shape and smell his smell. He pulls up my top and starts licking and stroking my breasts. I am getting very horny and start gasping and undoing his shirt buttons. He slowly moves his hand up my thigh and realizes that I have no knickers on and that my pussy is soft and wet and hot for him. I undo his trousers and take his dick in my hand, feeling the shape, the size. I start stroking his dick and balls in different ways to find out what turns him on most, and I get incredibly turned on by watching the expression on his face and listening to his groans.

He pushes up my skirt and presses his face into my pussy. He gently licks me with long, slow licks until I'm shaking all over and have to pull him off because I'm about to cum and want to cum with him inside me. He parts my lips, and I ease his dick inside me until it's all the way in, and it's filling me up and making me gasp with pleasure and then we both cum.

We imagine ourselves in an alleyway, on a beach, with our husband's best friend. We are close to orgasm, closer still, but wait! There are voices of people coming over the dunes about to discover us, naked, our orgasm almost upon us, their voices close, closer still and, dear Lord in heaven, we cum! We win! We live to complete another day against anti-sex rules. We triumph in the gamble of almost getting caught.

Faye

Faye, an educated thirty-one-year-old woman, having recently discovered masturbation, fantasizes being caught masturbating by her husband. Married for nine and a half years, monogamous for over eleven years, she's the daughter of divorced parents, has one child, a daughter, age four, and runs a small company. Of the five men she's been with, starting at age fifteen, three of them were long-term relationships.

This spring, I recently found out my husband was having cybersex via digital cameras and emails with women online. He never met up with these "women," but the act crushed me. I feel it was infidelity, but I know most think I'm being ridiculous. Either way, through therapy and much soul-searching, we decided to remain married, unless he messes up again. I don't want my daughter to see me as a doormat or, even worse, become one herself.

In January of this year, I discovered the joys of masturbation and sex toys. No, I didn't play with myself all day and ignore my husband. Until this January, I never experienced an orgasm. But I didn't know it! During sex, I felt my walls contract, and I would get damp and assumed this was an orgasm. My clit was always too sensitive to be touched. And I enjoyed sex…honest. My husband is a very giving man in bed and out, so I know I got more than enough foreplay.

*One night, I saw on cable a show where a woman got off using a "wand" on her clit. Up until then, a vibrator only numbed my cunt. So, I asked that night if we could try it—and **boom**! It happened! I was crying it felt so good. I was nervous about doing these things with* my husband—afraid I would hurt his ego (as he's very well-hung and such)—so, I felt embarrassed about asking to use my toys during sex. Then, his cyber thing happened and sex ceased. When we "healed," I realized maybe my new adventurous side might help us rather than hurt him. It has. He loves to watch me masturbate with my toys, and for the first time, he masturbated in front of me. I love it. Also, I ejaculate when I cum, and before reading up on the matter, I thought I was urinating. I can only g-spot when I have something (my husband's cock, hand, toy) penetrating me and a vibrator on my clit.

I never masturbated as a child. My parents were strict, and Dad was off having affairs most of their marriage. Mom raised me, never talking about sex. After their divorce, she became more open.

My fantasies are simple and kinda silly when compared to the details of others I read. I never fantasize about other men, just my husband.

In one fantasy, it's really snowy and cold out, and we have a hot tub in our backyard (which we don't). We relax in it as the snow falls and fuck like animals in it.

In another one, my daughter is not home, and I'm extremely horny. So, I lube up my favorite toy (a twisting, turning vibrating clit and vaginal machine—it's a must-have for any woman!) and get stark naked on our bed and begin to play. As I'm writhing around, I don't hear the door open. It's my husband, home from work early. He's an electrician and is filthy from work (plus that musky smell he gets from working hard, which I always love). I am embarrassed, but he's so turned on, he wipes his face with the bottom of his shirt, which he knows turns me on, and takes off his shirt and undoes his jeans, just enough to pull his cock out to jerk off in front of me. I finally cum, and he pulls my toy out, falls on me (with his jeans still on), and fucks me senseless.

It was The Great Architect's decision that the heart of sexual desire and the place where we urinate are the same, both of which we learned to control at the risk of losing mother's love.

The fantasies that some women invent begin with the absolute certainty that the *cloaca*—Latin for sewer—between our legs isn't a sewer at all but a garden of earthly delights. Wise men know this. He whose hot breath convinces us that our vagina is ambrosia is halfway home.

Meghan

Meghan's fantasy of her unusually well-endowed boyfriend has everything to do with his fantasies of her and his desire, lust, hunger of her vagina. The size of his penis would be inconsequential had he showed indifference.

I recently concluded a three-month relationship with a man who had the biggest penis I ever encountered. It was so big around that it would hardly enter me, and in fact, he could never penetrate me in any position other than the missionary one. (I am very tight.) On our first date, having met at a singles party, it was so obvious that we were very sexually attracted to one another, he reluctantly admitted to having a fantasy about me. I was not shocked or embarrassed but eager to hear about it, and he let me know in a few words that he had fantasized about eating me. (In fact, he fantasized constantly about eating me, even after we had begun having sex. He uses olive oil.) This made me so wild to experience it that after that date, I began to masturbate frequently, fantasizing about sex and oral sex with him. Within a few weeks, he ate me in the back of his van, which had curtains for privacy. It took another couple of weeks (in the van and in bed) before he could get his tremendous shaft all the way in without hurting me. That's when I found out that he screamed when he came.

Then, I discover that in spite of his having this gloriously huge penis, none of his previous lovers had ever paid a great deal of attention to it or had given him a real blow job, swallowing his cum. I loved to go down on that gigantic shaft, teasing him while he moaned and bit the pillows. Once, I gave him a blow job in his van after we had been to a restaurant, him helping by jerking it off as I sucked on it until he came in my mouth. This was so exciting for both of us! I thought about that often as well as how he screamed when he came. He was the best lover I ever had, and I know I was for him. He was more relaxed with his sexuality than any man I have ever known.

Years ago, when I began research on women's sexual fantasies, masturbation was a pleasure still untried by many women. Putting their hands between their legs was admitting failure at finding a man—meaning, failure as a "real woman." Add to that mother's warning that no "nice girl" went there. Pamela, a professional with an advanced degree, tells me, "I had sexual intercourse and was engaged before one night when I touched myself. I realized that I could give myself an orgasm…I immediately called my fiancé, ecstatic!"

Masturbation has now become for both sexes one of the handiest exercises in reducing tension, anxiety, and, yes, the iron grip of loneliness. I don't want to sound like I'm peddling a drug, but I must mention the *cosmetic* effect, the post-orgasmic blush to an otherwise pallid complexion, the easing of facial expression that invites others to say: "Have you been on vacation? You look wonderful!"

TOO MUCH OF A GOOD THING

Sometimes, I think the whole world is masturbating. Is that a good thing or bad? Does it say we are healthy for being free to own our bodies and find pleasure in them or is it a sad comment on our times, when so many people living alone prefer online chat to the sweetness and camaraderie of a physical partner?

Less than a hundred years ago, people would more likely die of starvation than obesity. The tables have turned. I read today that the government of Japan is now enforcing mandatory measuring of waistlines. Do the following two testimonials of Guido and Reese imply that at some point, the government may intervene and place restrictions on the time allowed to our masturbation?

Guido

Guido, a forty-six-year-old man, believes his sex life began when his mother started breast-feeding him as an infant. Though she stopped breast-feeding him at the age of two, he remembers at the age of four still wanting to suck her "pointed breasts," and because of his insistence, she finally conceded and agreed to it.

At the age of fourteen, I masturbated a lot, and my aunt caught me looking at a picture of a woman in her bra. My aunt said if I like bras, she would give me a bra to play with and produced a nice padded 36C cup. My aunt never told my mom, but I told her that I liked bras and tits, and she said that was natural.

Ever since then, I have masturbated with a bra. My mom was a 36B, and my aunt was eventually a 36D. I am single, but I have had plenty of girlfriends, but they always tire of me jerking myself off, and it's not long before we break up.

I still have fantasies of sucking a girl's tits full of milk, and while I'm sucking, she jerks me off, and I shoot my load in her bra, which she puts on and then rubs the cups so her milk and my juices mix.

One fantasy I have is with this girl, Talia, at her log cabin in the woods. When I arrive, she is dressed only in a bra and g-string panty and is wearing a cowgirl hat. She lights the candles, as they have cut her power, and we kiss on the couch. After passionately kissing, she gets up and takes off her panties. I am hard and take my shirt off and my denims and sit on the couch. She notices I have a big hard-on and then asks me to undo her bra, which I do. She has very pointed tits, and while we eat, her nipples get erect. After the main meal, she serves ice cream and chocolate wafers. I put some ice cream on her tits and lick it off. She pulls the g-string down in front and jerks me off, and I cum into her bowl of ice cream, which she mixes and then eats it all up.

Reese

Reese is a small-framed, sixty-five-year-old gay man who, through the miracle of the Internet, has become a "super-hot eighteen-year-old blonde chick with over thirty of the hunkiest boyfriends in the world." He grew up in a small Midwest town with a construction worker father, stay-at-home mother, and three macho older brothers who couldn't understand why he continuously stole his younger sister's dolls.

My first sexual experience happened when I was twelve with a neighborhood boy, Robby, my age but much larger. He threatened to tell the kids I was a cocksucker unless I agreed to give him a blow job.

It seemed like a strange way to prove my heterosexuality, but it began a love/hate relationship with bigger, aggressive men. I sometimes still masturbate to the memory of servicing Robby.

My favorite fantasy in high school was having the hottest gym coach coming into my room wearing only pajama bottoms while I'm in bed naked. He lies on top of me, begins kissing me, and says if I give him what he wants, he won't hurt me. I feel his hard cock grinding me. He pulls down his pajama bottoms, spreads my legs with his, then begins entering me. I would usually cum by then.

Most of the relationships I've had were with married men. They were fun at first, but by the mid-'70s, I accepted that love wasn't going to happen for me and in my mid-thirties developed an alcohol problem. After being arrested for lewd conduct during a drinking binge, I went into rehab, which is where I met my best friend. She's married to a well-known news personality, and I became his p.a. until I retired two years ago.

With so much free time, I'd been masturbating to the hot ads online, but then I placed an ad to attract just what I wanted. Kazzam! I became JH (short for Jim Hollander, the hottest boy in my high school in 1960). Jim Hollander was now looking for a muscle daddy to dominate him, someone much older, 25–45. Men were offering money, some persistently. But I'm not that kind of boy. Bi/gay men were all about sex, and I was too young and nervous to actually meet any of them.

Then, I became Kristy, a blonde, eighteen-year-old future pro cheerleader/supermodel/nursery school teacher looking for a strong, dominant, handsome older man, 25–45.

With the constant stream of pictures my nephew's wife emails of their super-hot daughter, Sam, I had plenty of proof I was real. The first picture I posted was just my head cut off above my cunning smile, revealing flowing blonde hair and a flawless body in a one-piece.

The response was awe-inspiring. Gorgeous hunks said they'd leave their wives for me. If my grandniece, Sam, only knew; I mean, she has a cute boyfriend in high school, but really.

My #1 boyfriend now is Dave, a pro football player. Being that I'm a cheerleader, I look up the rules online. We've been chatting for over a year. He keeps wanting to meet and talk on the phone. I finally had to admit that I'm only sixteen and can't talk because my father's very strict and checks my phone bill when he pays for it. Daddy would kill me and have Dave arrested if he ever found out. Dave's willing to wait. So am I. We keep sending each other pix. He's the hottest guy I've ever seen. I even got him to take some pix of his beautiful cock and send them to me. I can't tell you how many orgasms he's given me. Of course, I'm too shy to take x-shots. He can't wait till I'm old enough so he can hold me in his arms, and I tell him that will be incredible.

We're perfect for each other. Both our fantasies are about him dominating me. His weirdest one is where I'm surfing in Hawaii and a great white shark starts circling me. The shark starts pulling my surfboard, with me on it, out to sea. Seeing this, Dave rides in on his jet ski, jumps on the shark, and rips the shark's eyes out with his bare hands. Dave, covered in shark blood, takes me back to his beach hut, where I repay him for saving my life. My fantasies are often about him taking me in public places.

I know I now spend about as much time online as I do in the real world, anywhere from six to twelve hours a day. Lots of times I plan to go out but end up getting too involved chatting with several of my many gorgeous boyfriends.

I admit I'm a little jealous of Kristy. But when I'm her online, I love these studs trying to get me, sending any picture they can to seduce me. I love that they don't give up, even when they find out I'm underage and can't meet them for two years. They must be enjoying the fantasy, too. Not being able to have me probably really gets them going. My guess is, they don't want to blow the fantasy either. In reality, it's doubtful any of them would work with my grandniece. Sam's a great girl, but she's not Kristy.

Without the Internet, none of this would've ever happened. When I'm not online, I may be more depressed than when I was working. I have an addictive personality, but I know I'm not ready to stop. If it gets really bad, I'll probably go for help. But right now, I'm enjoying the ride.

Stefanie

When I asked Stefanie, a beautiful, Asian twenty-three-year-old, how the Internet has affected her sexual fantasies, she looked at me, askance. Many young people today are too young to have formed a sexual fantasy without the influence of the Internet.

I don't think I ever had a sexual fantasy till I went online. I was twelve. I didn't really think about sex. But after so many times of being told, "Don't go online—it's dangerous. You'll chat with perverts," of course, I had to go online. It was really hot looking at the men–meeting–women sites. Online, I almost only look at Asian men. But when I was sixteen, I dated a blond American guy with a Swedish background, and that was it—those are the kind of guys I like to date. For some reason, I still prefer masturbating to Asian men online, but I grew up in Northern California and really only get turned on to sex with Americans. I don't have an accent, and I like being with a guy who doesn't have one either. I love my parents, but I hate their accent. They sound like Asian tourists. It's such a turn-off thinking of having sex with a guy saying: "You likey? Is okay?"

In this day and age, besieged by mounting pressures to take charge of our lives, is it any wonder that so many people build to orgasm imagining that they are being taken, overwhelmed: "Beyond my control!" When did it start, this pervasive desire of both men and women to dream of being free of responsibility and to put in its place a "power greater than they demanding submission"?

As Rachel says: "I am so tired, so weary of responsibility and for everything and everyone. Oh, to be laid down and given pleasure! One more task, one more responsibility, and I'll scream! I need a power greater than my own to demand that I let go. I can't remember the last time I let some sweet somebody work me over. Oh, for the soothing orgasm, that sweet feeling building up—then letting go!"

As the pressures of our world increase, so do our desires to be coddled, pampered, controlled, disciplined, held once again in strong arms.

To Stefanie, her parents' accent makes them "the outsider," "the Asian tourists," threatening by association her own acceptance in her world, expulsion from the garden. To some degree, our parental figures are ever present. Because of our heightened sensitivity to what we perceive as their character flaws, we don't usually fantasize about our parents, but perhaps this is why, as turned off as Stefanie is to Asian accents, online she almost exclusively fantasizes of Asian men.

Our next four young men show that our desires are complex, a mix of submission and domination. Does the submissive partner never yearn to control or the dominant figure never long to be held/controlled/disciplined again under the loving care of mother and father? "Act like a man." "Don't cry like a girl." The boy's outward persona is shaped, carved by well-meaning caretakers. But our deepest desires haven't disappeared, only pushed farther into the recesses of our mind. We live in denial, hiding the fact that the need to be dominated, taken care of, is as natural as the desire for independence and control.

Steve

Steve, a seventeen-year-old, will soon be graduating from high school.

I've been masturbating since I was about thirteen or fourteen. My current practice is to straddle the lip of the toilet in my bathroom and bring the seat down and hook the thumb of my left hand around it so that it digs into the sensitive area just above my pubic hair. Then, with my right hand, I stimulate myself in time with my thrusts.

With my masturbation, my fantasies also evolved. My first fantasy was to visualize women from the Victoria's Secret online catalog. But then my fantasies started to get interactive. I visualized myself actually screwing women. My fantasies always seem to include an older woman. The reason for this is first off because that was the well of images I had to draw from, but there was another reason. I was about fifteen at the time. I had the day off from school and was just channel surfing when I came across a talk show. The topic was a seventeen-year-old kid who for the past four years had been having an affair with a forty-year-old woman. The idea so turned me on that I masturbated three times during the length of the broadcast.

One of my first fantasies was that I was doing some sort of work for a woman, and she asked me if I would like a drink, and we fell into talking. During our conversation, she starts showing off her body, such as stretching her arms far behind her head, or leaning far over so I can look down her shirt, or bending over to pick up something on the floor from the waist. This causes me to lose my train of thought several times while she goes on about her business as if nothing were happening. Finally, when I'm practically a pile of goo in my chair, she walks over and straddles me right there and asks me if I want her or not. We then proceed to fuck, either in her bed or on the kitchen floor.

The most recent fantasy of mine involves a teacher figure. I have been misbehaving in class and am told that she is very disappointed in me and that she is going to have to punish me. She then says that I must make reparations for the disturbance I have created in her class. These reparations come in the form of sexual slavery. I even have to take off her clothes in a certain manner. Sometimes, for spice, I imagine that the phone rings and that she has to talk to the principal of the school while I'm there thrusting my dick into her. One quick note: I'm pretty well-behaved in class, but if I knew that this was the punishment I would receive, I think I'd be tempted to act up a bit.

Rory

Rory, a bisexual man from a "fairly liberal family, even by Western standards," is a British Asian citizen. After several suicide attempts, his father, a doctor, got him into therapy, and he has had treatment for four years. He is no longer suicidal and is just about ready to "come out" and tell his parents he is bisexual.

My gay feelings are much stronger than my "straight" ones, though my interest in women has grown. I've had one brief relationship with a man of my own age.

A lot of my gay feelings involve a father figure. I used to show my hard-on to my dad and ask if it was normal and "accidentally" show him myself naked. He's a pediatrician and sees a lot of confused adolescents. He was understanding, but he's very mild and inhibited, with bouts of clinical depression that have brought my parents' marriage to nothing. These exhibitions always turned me on, and I'd always masturbate afterward. I've had fantasies of anal sex with him, both ways.

I fantasize a lot about meeting a man in his mid-thirties, a real role model: tall, strong, Irish accent, blond, uninhibited—he hugs and kisses his men friends in the straightest way imaginable. The attraction doubles the second he says he has a son almost my age. I want to be straight. I want to be a husband and father. And I want him because he's these things. It's his straightness I desire.

I imagine I am Brendan's son. His wife is nowhere around—divorced probably.

I'm seventeen, and we've often talked about sex and seen each other naked all the time and wrestled. I imagine lying down next to him when he's dozing. We're both in shorts and nothing else. He wakes up and puts his arms around me and smiles. I put my face against his neck and kiss him. I look at his muscles, firm, strong, but not huge. This is a man like me, strong but vulnerable as well—firm but tender. His hair is in a ponytail, and I loosen it. His big brown eyes are staring down at me, and when I kiss his chest, he sees what I want.

He has decades more experience than me, and it shows as he caresses me. He uses his palm or his fingers together. He doesn't use one fingertip on its own—this isn't teasing sex; this is more like hugs and slow, soft cuddle. I'm not the skinny guy. I really am muscular or perhaps pudgy. But either way, there is rich, warm flesh and enough to supply lots of contact between our bodies.

Early afternoon sunlight slants through the window as we kiss, using our tongues to explore each other. The hair on the back of his arms is golden in the buttery light, and a chain around his neck dangles in front of his nipples as they become harder and a little rosy.

He calls me "my baby boy" in a quiet voice, his low, rich Irish voice. Soon, I move down to his cock and use slow, relaxed movements to make him harder. He lies on his back, his hands in my hair. He stiffens, his back arches, and his breathing gets heavier. I can feel his cock, hard as stone, but warm and pulsing in my mouth. My mouth floods with saliva as I feed on Dad. And soon he groans, his head thrown back, and he floods my mouth with his milky manhood. I swallow and crawl up to his face again, and we kiss, slow and soft. I'm hard, and soon his hands are on my back, and I'm kissing the top of his head as he kneels in front of me, his knees wide apart, as he takes me, his son, deep into himself, with broad generous strokes of his tongue. Soon I cum, giving him the love-gift he passed on to me a moment ago.

Danny

Danny is a twenty-two-year-old "mostly straight" white man. His father is a liberal/conservative; liberal in most of his thinking but conservative when it comes to sex, barely acknowledging it exists. His mother, on the other hand, is a lesbian with feminist views. Sexual politics are always a discussion with her. His adult fantasies are of a wide variety, most of them straight, some of them bi or homosexual, and a few of them relating to children and childhood. He often masturbates to thoughts of women fingering themselves and has masturbated several times with young women friends who were as curious as he was about the opposite sex's masturbation practices.

One time, I answered an ad in the newspaper for "British school discipline." I was twenty-one at the time, but I wanted to live out my childish fantasy to the fullest, so I shaved my body from my navel to my ankles, giving myself the young boy look. I walked up to the door of the house wearing shorts and a T-shirt, exposing my hairless legs. A stern-looking man in his fifties ushered me in. When I entered his living room, he ordered me to undress. I pulled off my T-shirt and my socks and then moved to my shorts. I anticipated the look on the man's face when he would see my hairless bottom and penis. I pulled off my underwear. He marched me downstairs to a bedroom where I lay across his lap while he spanked me with his hand and then a hairbrush. Later, he bent me over a bed and strapped me with a belt and then spanked me with a large paddle. My buttocks were just throbbing after that, but the whole time my penis was erect, and I was close to orgasm. Afterward, he rubbed cream on my bottom and stroked my penis while he told me about other "boys" he had spanked and what had turned them on. I still think of this often, fantasizing that a woman is there with me, forced to watch before enduring a spanking herself.

Brent

Brent is a twenty-year-old college student. A neighbor in her forties asked him and his friend in for some sex play after making passes at them from her balcony. Unfortunately, her husband appeared before they could do anything.

Therefore, I only have a fantasy, which I jack off to all the time. It goes like this: My friend and I begin to slowly undress this gorgeous woman. She has a really nice tan and is wearing a string bikini. My friend and I slowly begin to kiss her all over her entire body from head to toe. Suddenly, she begins to give us commands and tells us we must obey her. "Suck my pussy through my bikini," she tells me. Then, she tells my roommate that she wants to "see a show" before we begin undressing her. "I want both of you to fuck me, but first I want to watch you play with each other." She then instructs us to pull off our swimsuits. "I want you to lick each other and explore your bodies." At first, we protest, but we're starting to get pretty turned on watching her fingering her pussy and knowing what's ahead when we get to have all of her. I notice my dick getting pretty hard, and my roommate already has a full-fledged erection. The woman tells me: "Sit down on the bed and suck your roommate's cock while he stands over you. I want to see you suck that big thing. Make him really hard." Then, she tells my roommate to do the same to me. I become really erect as he puts his mouth over my long six-inch rod.

"Now that you're really turned on, I want both of your hard dicks in me at the same time." She pushes me on the bed and jumps on my dick, putting it in her sopping wet pussy, while instructing my roommate to put his dick into her tight ass that she just finished lubricating. We eagerly comply. "Now I want both of you to fuck me hard. Fuck me like you've never fucked before. Make me feel good." Then, she tells us how horny she has gotten just watching us the last few weeks and how it's "payback time" for her.

Suddenly, the woman's husband walks in and sees us both humping her at the same time. She tells her husband that she is enjoying herself and loves having two young cocks at the same time and that she's not stopping for anything. Her husband is very surprised but excited at the same time, and he begins unbuttoning his blue jeans, revealing his bulging dick under his briefs. He begins jacking off just watching us. Suddenly, the woman begins to moan so loudly, it's deafening. "I'm getting what I want. Fuck me hard!" At about that point, my roommate and I both are about ready to cum as the woman begins to writhe up and down on the bed near orgasm. Her husband moves closer, and we all scream with pleasure as he shoots wads of his cum all over us. Afterward, my roommate and I and her husband softly stroke the woman and caress her with body oil until she falls asleep.

DON'T ASK ME—I'M ONLY YOUR PARENT

Our later sexual activity will always have a relevance to the early years when we were alone with our bodies. No one ever said our genitals were a beautiful place. We were taught to brush our teeth so that they would serve us a lifetime, to stand up straight, and not to strain our eyes. But no one said a word about the care, respect, and maintenance of the springboard of our sexual feeling. Why care for a place that has no value, a place that we females can never get clean enough?

We wonder why adolescents risk pregnancy and disease, why HIV is increasing in young gay men. Stealth and risk have become integral to our orgasm. Many young women today think no better of their genitals than we did thirty years ago. How different would we be had our parents been open and honest with us, taught us to be proud of our genitals, and, yes, *meant* what they said?

Heather

Heather is a twenty-six-year-old white mother of three girls, ages three, four, and six. She was married to her first husband, an abusive alcoholic, for five years and has been married for three years to a loving second husband. Raised by conservative grandparents, with a reticent attitude toward sex, she lost her virginity at the age of thirteen to a boy she was dating. She didn't use protection, the pill, until she was fourteen, miscarried at seventeen, and, similar to Susannah, became pregnant and married at nineteen.

I was a big dater and very active after I was raped at age fifteen. I figured I was never going to fall in love and no one was going to love me because of the rape. So, I began to date just about anyone who asked, and if sex was mentioned, it usually was done. I also dated mostly guys who were a few years older. My first husband was ten years older, and sex was great till the bottle took over. After that, it was like being raped all over again. I began masturbating then, which is when my fantasies began.

I met my current and hopefully last husband (four years older) while I was going through my divorce. After our first date, we wanted to make love and after two weeks couldn't keep our hands off each other. So, my girls and I moved in with him. He travels at least once a year, and during those times, I masturbate fantasizing about him being with me.

My most recent fantasy has to do with where he is right now: I'm dressed in a harem costume complete with crotchless panties, and I'm in his dorm. He thinks I'm at home in the States. He comes back to find me waiting for him. I have drawn him a warm bath and have massage oil waiting for him. He is in a state of shock but allows me to undress him even though he has a million questions. I kiss his body as I undress him, and since we have been apart for so long, his penis rises to attention quickly. I tell him to get in the bath, and he does. I wash him, stopping to give his male member extra attention. After his bath, I dry him off, again kissing his whole body as I do so. I tell him to lie on his belly and give him a massage, then make him roll over onto his back. I massage his chest and legs, avoiding his penis, which really makes him crazy. I then begin to massage his penis with my mouth and tongue, first slowly, and then lick his balls in between. Then, I spring back to his penis, first slow and then with a quickening pace. Before he can cum, he has to please me, too, so he proceeds to lick my clit and finger-fuck my pussy. He alternates fingers with his tongue till I have orgasms a number of times. Then, when I can't take any more, I make him enter me with my legs over his shoulders. While he is pumping in and out, he sucks on my breasts (which still have breast milk). We finally cum together, and, boy, are there fireworks! Afterward, we bathe each other and just lay together wrapped in a huge towel.

THANKS FOR THE MEMORIES

In spite of our total dependence on our caretakers, we defy them to follow eros, the good feeling. And we keep defying them. But here's the real glory. We don't just pursue eros; we take the anti-sex warnings from the nursery and turn them around, spin them into gold—as in a fairy tale.

Arthur

Arthur is a thirty-nine-year-old man, raised in England, First Class Honors degree and law degree, now living in America.

At sixteen, my mother examined my underpants one fine summer's day for the presence of semen. She suspects I've been masturbating. (I have, for years. But this time, I fool her—no semen on the pants. She draws a blank.) Some months later, though, she barges into my bedroom and catches me at it. Big Scene. Fireworks. Me reduced to a quivering puddle of guilt. She tells me I'm a "filthy little bastard" and threatens to kick me out of the house.

Ever since I've started masturbating, around age ten or eleven, I've done so lying on my stomach. (Look, ma, no hands.) Now that I'm single again, I do so at least once a day, sometimes twice. Occasionally, I get off online—especially with an imaginative, sensitive, intelligent woman on the other end—in which case, I take off everything. Like some women, who even take off their earrings and wristwatches before masturbating or making love, there's a delicious feeling of total abandon, which comes from being absolutely naked. Sometimes, at work, I jerk off—discreetly— face down on the couch, hiding my naked buns under a blanket in case of any unexpected interruptions.

In one of my fantasies, I imagine myself as a biology teacher in an all-girls boarding school in France. Sitting in the front row is a beautiful dark-eyed girl. She's Lolita—the classic Nabokovian "nymphet"—an arresting combination of guile and innocence. Suddenly, she gets up and leaves the classroom without a word. I wait. Ten, twenty, thirty minutes elapse, but she doesn't come back. Concerned, I decide to investigate. The door is ajar. I peer round, and—sure enough—there she is, lying flat on her back, her head propped up by a pillow.

Somehow she's gotten hold of a stethoscope. It's the old-fashioned kind, the kind that makes you shiver, with the metal bulb, which feels cold on your skin. Very slowly she unbuttons her top, button by button, and draws the material aside. Her tummy is as smooth and brown as her arms, her navel flawless, concave, and—somehow— endearingly innocent.

At this point, she realizes that someone's watching. Instead of trying to cover up, she puts down the stethoscope, reaches over to the drawer of her night stand, and takes out a bottle of baby oil. One drop at a time, she fills her navel until it overflows and trickles down her sides and onto the sheets. Then, she starts to rub the oil in. One hand moves to her swollen nipples, while the other starts to work furiously at her tight little clit. "Close the door, monsieur," she whimpers. "I want you to make me cum."

I undress and tell her to put her hands behind her head. I start to lick her nipples and nibble them gently between my teeth. Then, I work my way down her stomach, toward her navel, which she thrusts up to meet the tip of my tongue. At last, I start on her clit.

By this time, she's writhing and groaning, begging me to fuck her. I stop and tell her to lie completely still. She whimpers, a combination of defiance and frustration. I fetch a lamp and shine it directly onto her tummy so that I can see the web of silvery hairs and the delicious contours of her abdominal muscles beneath. And then I'm inside her. Her pussy is so tight that it takes all the strength of will I can muster not to cum on the spot. As she moves closer to climax, her body buckles, and her stomach muscles quiver and harden. I lick her ear and tell her that I want her to watch. She glues her eyes to the tip of my cock, wet with precum and inches from orgasm, waiting for it to shoot out its liquid fire all over her belly. As I cum, she arches her back and lets out an unearthly scream as her own climax erupts deep inside her and rubs the stuff round and round, coating her belly and inner thighs. The contrast—my white seed on her brown skin—is too startling to put into words.

"MARRIAGE IS LIKE THE MIDDLE EAST—THERE'S NO SOLUTION"
Or Is There?

Married sex often becomes a disappointment...unless we accompany it with fantasy.

Manny

I was infatuated with my wife. I loved the way her body felt and the softness of her breasts and nipples. We enjoyed sexual intercourse very much. Now that we're older, our sexual activity has dropped off. I've resumed masturbating to satisfy my male urge.

It seems I get my fantasies from where I least expect them. I never looked forward to going to the dentist, but last week, I had my teeth cleaned, and the dental hygienist was a cute young woman dressed in a soft pullover sweater and white slacks. She laid me back in the chair until I was horizontal, and she took a chair at my shoulder. She rested her arm on my chest, and at times, I could feel her breast pushed against my head. Sometimes, when I opened my eyes, her boob was just a couple of inches away from me.

I started thinking it would be nice if I could take my hand and put it on her back or how it would feel if she didn't have a bra on. I thought about running my hand under her sweater and moving up to her bra and unfastening it. Then, I would run my hand over her tit and feel her nipple. I could tell she was beginning to become aroused, and she moved so I could play with her other tit.

She would stop her cleaning for a few moments to rest, and she would smile and move her hand down to my semi-hard cock and gently rub it. Then, she'd say, "I'll be finished with your teeth in a few minutes, and we'll move on to other things." As she rests again, she unzips my trousers and reaches in to find my cock and gives it a few strokes.

She moves back just a little and takes off her sweater, and her loose bra falls off her breasts. She tells me I can suck them, and she moves close so I can suck each of them. She then says, "That's enough, let me finish." My hands fondle her breasts as she finishes up.

The door is already closed because this is a special dentist office catering to men and offering some "extras" along with the dentistry (lighter dental work). Sometimes, the hygienist is topless as she begins her work. She now unfastens my pants and pulls them down, along with my shorts. She moves right in and begins to suck my cock as she gently fondles my balls. I move my hand to her cunt (she's already taken off her clothes), and I start to rub her clit.

Her mouth is moving up and down my cock as I get harder, and I start to feel myself nearing orgasm. I have two fingers in her cunt and am rubbing her clit. I can tell she is getting close to orgasm, too.

I can no longer hold back, and I shoot a big load in her mouth, and my fingers bring her to a climax, too. She smiles at me and moves to kiss me on the lips and lets some of my cum into my mouth. I like the taste.

She tells me it's time for her next patient, and she'll look forward to my next cleaning.

Back in reality, I now look forward to mine.

WHY PAY WHEN YOU CAN STEAL?

I once thought if I, Nancy, was rhapsodic over masturbation one more time in my writing, my mother would disown me. Actually, she and I went through our rapprochement when I wrote *My Mother, My Self*, the book that immediately followed *My Secret Garden*. I've always found it fascinating, and absolutely right, that the thought occurred to me to write about mothers and daughters as I was writing the last page of *My Secret Garden*. "Why are women so cut off from their sexual selves? Who would want the world to believe that women don't have sexual fantasies?" I asked. And answered: "Mother."

I still feel a certain frisson when I write the word *masturbation*, almost as if I were breaking the law. That is how I felt the first time I touched myself and felt the mix of Heaven and Hell. I assume, even hope, that I will never outgrow the excitement of stolen sex, on which I was raised.

We masturbate in spite of Mother, God, and Country. A defining, if not defiant, act. It is rare when we find anyone who, unsolicited, approves, says it's OK.

We have no idea that this surreptitious hold on the forbidden place between our legs tells us how we will feel about our bodies for the rest of our lives. Stolen sex will always be the sweetest fruit on the tree.

Tony

Tony is a thirty-seven-year-old African American head teacher in a primary school and was raised in a conservative family where both parents were reticent to talk about sex.

My earliest sexual experience was at age four or five when I found myself under a large packing crate with an older boy of about seven or eight. He was skinning back his foreskin while I and a boy my age watched him. I can still recall the odor and how wicked and exciting it all seemed. I remember shortly after this wanting to pee outside *the house, and this had some vague connection for me with the sexual activity under the box, but I wasn't able to work it out. My mother found me peeing outside and was pretty horrified.*

The next specifically sexual activity took place when I was about nine or ten. A friend who was about a year older than me was given a soft porn magazine by his father while I was standing in their kitchen. The mother was also there, and she just smiled as he opened the pages, and we both saw a topless woman standing in front of a haystack. The sight of her naked breasts (probably the first I had seen) and the fact that both parents approved *was to become a powerful image for me. It was astonishing. I idealized this family, and have constructed a number of fantasies around them.*

I had my one and only sex education lesson from a teacher I now think is gay. He told the class the mechanics of male masturbation and likened the orgasm to "a huge and wonderful sneeze." The next chance I had, I tried it out. I remember it was a Saturday morning, and I was lying in bed at home. At first, there was no sensation as I stroked my cock, but I soon felt a sensation that grew and grew. After about five minutes, this feeling developed into a buzzing, tingling surge, and I came. To my surprise, there was no emission. I was overcome with delight and an almost euphoric sense of well-being. My family was a fairly strict Baptist one in which there was a strong taboo on sexuality and related talk, *never mind* activity. *At this moment, I also had a sense of relief that I hadn't done anything "wrong." Without ejaculating, it didn't count as a sin. But after a few more times, I ejaculated and continued* to from then on. I realized it had moved into the guilt-laden phase, but I was also fascinated by the sight of the white, hot, sticky liquid I was able to produce.

I called on my friend with the porn magazines, but his mom said he was out. She was wearing a thin housecoat, and I could see the outline of her breasts quite clearly. She asked me in to wait and sent me up to his room. As soon as I was in there, I went for his collection of magazines. Leafing through one, I started to get aroused and pushed my hand into my jeans to stroke my thickening cock. I dropped my pants and heard a noise downstairs. My friend came bounding into the room before I had time to zip up or hide the magazines. He just grinned when he saw what I'd been doing. "Feel like a wank myself," he said and took his jeans down, pulled out his very long cock, and started going at it. I heard his mom coming upstairs and was almost paralyzed with panic. What if she saw us? But he didn't seem to care. He was staring at his magazine and breathing very loudly when his mom walked in. Neither was shocked. In fact, his mom stopped and looked quite proudly at her son's cock and smiled at me, holding my own temporarily wilted cock, before demurely leaving, closing the door behind her.

One fantasy has me in my friend's room on my own, waiting for him. I get out his magazines and just stroke myself when I hear his mom coming up the stairs. She walks along to her room, humming almost absentmindedly. She then calls my name softly, asking if I could help her for a minute. I feel very turned on at not being caught and her proximity. I walk into her room. She's sitting on the bed with one leg down, the other on the bed. She has stockings on and is adjusting her garter. "Which do you think is best?" She holds out two bras: one black and the other white. I can hardly breathe. She then opens her housecoat and stands up. I don't know what to do. Her breasts are large, heavy but not drooping. She takes my hand and places it on her boob, smiling. "Have you done this

*before?" she asks. I can only shake my head. "Lick and kiss," she says.
I lean forward and take her nipple in my mouth. She's breathing deeply
and is clearly turned on. I lick, tease, and suck on one, then the other,
backward and forward, with my cock straining for release.*

*She undoes my jeans and sweeps them down. She sits on the bed and
looks at my stiff cock. Her face is one of concentration and lust. She
takes me in her hand and gently pulls me toward her mouth. She kisses
the purple crown and then opens wide and very slowly sinks her mouth
over my cock. I think I'm going to cum there and then, but she very
slowly moves her head backward and forward, sucking quite hard on
my cock and drawing the most wonderful buzzing feelings from me.*

*She stops, lies back on the bed, and tells me to get on it with her. She
slips her bottoms off, and I get on. She then straddles me with her knees
on either side of my head. She lowers her mouth onto my cock and her
pussy onto my lips. I've never seen one, and here I'm eating the most
delightful, musky-fragranced pussy. She's sawing her pelvis back and
forth and heavily lubricating. I push my tongue well in, swirl it around,
and before I know it, both she and I are cumming noisily and profusely.
There's a noise downstairs, and I freeze. She makes no move as the
person comes upstairs. It's her husband. He just puts his head round
the door, smiles at us both, and says, "Hi."*

⚜

We girls all knew the boy grows up handling his penis, for
no other reason than to urinate. And even if he doesn't bring
himself to erection, the penis has a mind of its own. Roy, a handsome man, says, "I spent a lot of time scratching my head when
I was eleven over what the Boy Scout Handbook meant by 'noc-
turnal emission.' Then came a dream in which I remember tall

blondes in high heels. They were naked otherwise, and I could see their titties and hairy pussies. And I woke up with the crotch of my briefs soaked with something warm and sticky. I thought I'd wet the bed and so I told no one. I didn't really know what was up until I was in the ninth grade."

He wakes in the night with a wet dream. When you think about it, the boy's body is teaching him—literally—precisely what turns him on, what his favorite aphrodisiac is, and just when and where he wants it. What a marvelous tool. Is it any wonder that young girls—myself included—envy this magical wand of the lad that allows him to stand and pee? Oh, yes, when very young, I tried it and thoroughly drenched my socks and shoes.

Do I romanticize the boy's sexual coming of age? God knows, I wanted to be a boy when I was ten, stood at the end of the diving board, alone one summer eve and tried to pee a high arc into the water. Yes, I envied the boy his freedom, until a short time later when I didn't want to be him but to hold him, be held by him. No longer wanting my own penis but to feel his pressed against me, precisely against that sensitive button that rocketed me to the moon when he held me very close in the dance.

DOES PRACTICE MAKE PERFECT?

Kris

Kris is a forty-three-year-old financial advisor. Both he and his wife lost interest in sex about halfway into their marriage. It had become "routine." They both felt, "Why bother?" For the last ten years of the marriage, until his divorce, his only sexual activity was masturbation.

When I started dating again, primarily meeting women online, I was so used to masturbating I found I couldn't orgasm inside them. I'd have to pull out and jerk off on her. It was very frustrating and unsatisfying. A few mentioned that I was like a porn star. I couldn't tell them that their vaginas just weren't working like my hand.

I usually fantasize taking a beautiful woman, one I've chatted with online, but what always brings me to instant orgasm is thinking of a female bodybuilder taking me, using me to satisfy herself. I try not to masturbate to that fantasy too much because if I get used to it, it makes it harder for me to orgasm inside the woman I'm seeing.

I was finally able to cum again in a woman by changing the way I masturbate, shaping my hand more like a vagina and fucking it. I also learned not to jerk off to completion in the morning if I thought I might be having sex that night. I know—"Duh!" The reason I masturbated once in the morning and once at night was more fear of "use it or lose it" than of just being horny. There's so little we're taught about sexual function. If we have some muscle ailment, it's the most natural thing in the world to discuss it with your colleagues, but I've never heard anyone say in pre-board-meeting meeting chat, "You know, I think I'm jerking off too much, and that's why I'm not able to cum inside a woman."

MASTURBATION AND THE CURSE

I was thirteen before I knew that the boy masturbates. How could he not when his penis stands, demanding attention? But it isn't just the design of women's bodies that distances us from practicing masturbation. Because we are the same sex as the woman who bore and raised us, she is the unavoidable model of how to be, act, how to do and feel almost everything. Unless of course we take her as a negative role model, as often as not out of spite, as in, "Very well, Mommy, if you don't love me then I'll do and be everything different from you."

Just when a lad's been looking for a way to free himself from mother's hold on him, his own body points the way. In an insightful and evocative letter, Nelson, who was raised by a single mother, comments: "It is a cycle. A boy is raised by a woman. He becomes her best friend or, as in my case, the little husband. It took a long time before I could have a serious relationship with a girl. I had to finally detach myself from my mother." He and Mom meet all of each other's emotional needs, but, of course, that time occurs when his sexual needs assume a dominant position. He can't conceive of Mom in those terms, but since Mom is meeting all of his emotional needs, he is really not able to be emotionally involved with a girl.

As adolescents, boys, naturally separating from their mothers, begin to "hang out" in secretive places where competitive games involving penises can be played. It's still one of the few "No Girls Allowed!" zones. The locker room will reinforce solidarity. It's a guys-only place where naked cocks of all sizes and shapes "hang" together.

What a symbol for separation—the penis! With every stroke, he is defying Mom and simultaneously reinforcing his own separate identity.

Women often wonder why the man, fully grown, is so devoted to what lies between his legs. Years go by, and grown men still eye each other's cocks in the locker room. Of course, he may want a woman to hold it, but he's been holding it, first to urinate and then to masturbate, for most of his life.

The camaraderie we women had in our youthful sleepovers gets tossed by the competition that begins with adolescence, when every girl finds herself bleeding once a month—alas, not a ritual bolstering solidarity.

Menstruation, earlier these years than ever, reinforces the girl's tie to the woman who bore her. Whatever gains in separation we've attained so far can be diminished in the absolute replication of mother. Menstrual blood further soils the damp "cloaca" between our legs. And it happens at the same time when a girl is first drawn romantically and sexually to boys who are eager to touch "that place," to see it.

Whatever curiosity the girl may have had about her vagina is put into question. Now that she is menstruating, she may feel more than ever the desire to arouse herself, but her feelings about "that place" have changed. Her masturbatory fantasies are likely to become filled by imaginary scenes of being forced, overpowered into spreading her legs and succumbing to the boy-man's brave exploration of "the sewer."

A lot has happened in the past thirty years, but are mothers today that much more aware of the healthy benefits of masturbation, not just pleasure but responsibility? How can you expect a child to grow up taking care of her body if she harbors a "sewer"?

It's tough for young women to think well of the vagina when one day, out of the blue, and just about the time we've got everything under control, there is blood coming out of "that place." What if we soil our clothes in public with blood? So many women take menstruation as a time to stop touching themselves, bringing themselves to orgasm, when the time couldn't, in fact, be better. Bleeding once a month is power; so is masturbation.

Betsy

Betsy, a fifteen-year-old high school student whose mother has never spoken to her about sex, sometimes stays home from school, sick, due to menstruation. All her sexual knowledge comes from romance novels, to which she masturbates on a regular basis. But the "heroines never menstruate"; therefore, for them, it's a nonissue. She says she wants to wait until marriage for sex because it has to be with someone who won't mind if she bleeds.

My cousin introduced me to romance novels, and I've been addicted ever since. When I read sex novels, I get very aroused. I climax from reading them and masturbating. I only cum if I massage my clitoris. I also become aroused when I read about human/animal sex. I'm not sure why.

I don't usually need my own fantasies because I read other people's. One of my old ones is people on a cruise ship as a sexual getaway with orgies, homosexual and heterosexual versions of it. A recent fantasy is a woman who is addicted to sex, and when her husband is at work, she has all kinds of guys (high school jocks to plumbers to neighbors) over to have sex. It could be with one guy or a marathon with several.

I believe masturbation is a form of self-gratification and is basically therefore a sin. But I like it. It's sort of addictive because I can't stop, though I know I should be doing more important things.

Through recent interviews, I've found that a woman masturbating may not be as appealing to men as it was thirty years ago. Perhaps, because of the Internet, it's now so accessible. Or that competing with women in the workplace has taken some of the blush off the rose. But when the mating dance does begin, most males expect that we are as fond of our vaginas as they are of their penises. What a jolt to learn the reason we are reluctant to accept his adoration of what lies between our legs isn't because we prize it so dearly but instead disparage the sight and smell of it.

How did it get such a bad name, touching this place between our legs? It's clean, easy, cheap, takes the edges off anxiety, and, yes, teaches us that our orgasm is our responsibility, that our sexuality resides within ourselves and isn't a gift that another person controls. Where did anti-masturbatory rules come from? In an age such as ours, plagued by violence, drug addiction, sexually transmitted diseases, it should be made a law that parents encourage their children to do what is natural.

The individual's need to be in control has accelerated as the world grows more chaotic. I am not weighing erotic pleasure opposite today's disasters, simply suggesting that what God gave us might be reassessed and acknowledged as the gifts they are.

The vagina has come into its own in recent years, and nothing has been more helpful than masturbation. How can you denigrate a place that can give so much pleasure with so little effort?

A man rejoices, "Women really do love sex, just like me!" He is overjoyed, full of surprise and gratitude at the idea of women enjoying masturbation, that a woman would be so hot—like him—and would reach orgasm simply by putting her hands between her legs—like him. But nothing convinces a man that women enjoy sex as much as when she initiates the sex—actually lays him down and does him.

CONFESSIONS OF A BOY TOY

Ryan

The son of Irish Catholic parents and a professor of literature, Ryan writes in great and exquisite detail of his "sunrise" fantasy with his girlfriend, who is studying art in Venice, and "sunset" fantasy with a woman who is off-limits.

My fantasy in the afternoon involves a young Latin American girl who lives in my same apartment building. I'll call her Martina. She's studying art and photography at the same university where I teach. Incidentally, this prevents me from asking her out. I am completely intoxicated by her. When I see her pull up in her car, I'll often change into my running shorts and go out my door, descending the stairs as she goes up. We often exchange greetings. A few times, she has even knocked on my door, seeking advice, usually something related to her studies.

In my fantasy, I see her pull up in her car. I take my shirt off. (I'm in excellent physical shape—blond, tanned, well-toned body—so why not try to seduce her?) I see that she's depressed and ask her what's wrong. She tells me her model cancelled on her the last minute and her portfolio is due tomorrow. What model? I ask her. She blushes slightly, saying she needs some photographs of a male. Why don't you photograph me, I suggest. She throws her arms round my neck, telling me, could I be serious? I say, sure, why not? Then, she looks past me, biting her lip, her dark hair falling past her eyes, before she looks into my eyes, and almost whispers, "Will you model for me—nude?"

I tell her to let me think about it while I run a few miles. As I run, I have a hard-on the whole time. When I get back to the apartment, there's a note on my door: "Ryan, I will always be in your debt. Martina." I go to her door, and just as I get ready to knock, she answers, handing me a glass of white wine. She's playing jazz, and she's wearing a kind of kimono. I can see her nipples peeking out slightly to the side of the silky material as she leans over to pick up her camera from a table. She tells me she'll step out of the room a minute while I get out of my clothes. My hard-on has gone down, but I'm afraid it will return when Martina re-enters. I think about baseball and football, fishing, anything to put heat out of my loins. I step out of my gym shorts and wait. Martina comes back into the room, smiles, and compliments me for having a sexy body. She says my body is much sexier than the guy who cancelled on her in the last minute. She begins snapping photos, asking me to try to move to the rhythm of the music. She keeps saying, "Beautiful, baby, beautiful," as she snaps photo after photo from a variety of angles. She then says she wants me to lean facedown on her bed, as she photographs me from behind, telling me the whole time I have one sexy bottom.

She tells me to stand in the middle of the room as she opens the shades and lets the soft sunlight into the room. She wants me wet and asks me not to move as she rubs mineral water into my hair, brushing her pelvis up against my cock (now hardening). She then towel-dries my hair slightly, her tits and hard nipples now protruding out of her kimono, nearly touching my lips as she rubs me on tiptoes. By now I'm completely hard and throbbing against her pelvis. She then squirts baby lotion over my chest and buttocks, rubbing the oil all over my body, sometimes teasing my cock as she runs her palm lightly over my thighs. She begins photographing me, telling me I have a delicious cock, that I'm as sexy as Michelangelo's David, and that if I don't cum, she's going to be very nice to me.

She lets the kimono fall to the floor, and her cunt is absolutely beautiful, with her dark moist pubis in front of me. She tells me, pointing to her lithe body, that this is all mine for modeling for her. I rush to her, embrace her legs, and lick her thighs before circling her dripping clit with my tongue, taking in her delicious scent, before plunging my tongue deeper, licking and sucking, and she writhes with pleasure. She whimpers with delight and then has a shattering orgasm, causing her to buckle and fall to the floor. I won't let her go. I begin sucking her breasts, kissing her neck, turning her on her belly, kissing her peach-shaped ass. I then fuck her with slow gentle strokes, caressing her wet vaginal lips with the tip of my cock, before slowly sliding it into her deeper, with long rhythmic strokes, sticking my index finger up her tight ass.

She begins screaming and moaning as I finally let out a tremendous flow of semen deep into her cunt. I turn her over, let her kiss her own juices off my lips, and then she moves down on me, lapping my belly and taking my once again hard dick into her mouth, her lipstick-coated lips leaving a ring around my shaft as I have another orgasm. She then tells me to leave, handing me some money, and tells me she might want me to model again for her soon.

I listen to my contributors in this book, read the headlines in the morning paper, the Internet's endless coverage of everything, and wonder how today's world affects eros. Growing up now, physical and emotional boundaries ever expanding, a sureness of life vanishing, we live in a kind of chaos. I am deeply moved by the self-portraits of young people in this book. Can we be surprised when they speak of masturbatory fantasies of torture and punishment, both physical and emotional?

We no longer need a partner to "complete" ourselves. Aside from anatomical differences, men and women duplicate one another, do the same jobs, and raise children without the opposite sex. Before we had the answer to everything—thanks to the Internet—we cosseted the mysteries, the unknowns that were aroused by sex. Without the crucial differences between the sexes, we say to ourselves, "I don't need anyone. I am complete unto myself."

Masturbation has never been more prevalent. What has diminished is romantic music, the feelings of longing, the excruciating sense of "I'll die if you leave me, if I don't see you soon, if you don't hold me and arouse in me that deep sense of urgency."

Is it any wonder that fantasies of being *made* to succumb and forced to lay down are so prevalent?

JANE TAKES TARZAN

Sam

Sam, a thirty-two-year-old, handsome Latin American, happened to walk in on a neighbor couple's hot sex as a teenager. As the woman was on top of the man, he perceived her to be dominant, taking him. Excited by what he saw, he immediately went home to masturbate and now has a plethora of fantasies in his arsenal of women who are in a position of power over him sexually. In contrast to Ryan, he is not just a sex symbol but a powerful man overtaken by an even more powerful woman.

My current fantasies tend to be very well-developed and quite involved. I am usually a character of popular folklore. For example, in one, I am Tarzan, King of the Jungle. I am handsome, well-built, and wear only a skimpy leopard-skin bikini. I rule by virtue of my strength and fighting ability. One day, some of the male natives tell me of rumors about a woman named Sheena who rules another part of the jungle. They say that they are finding it increasingly difficult to control their women because it is said that this Sheena is coming to confront and defeat Tarzan and will then establish a society dominated by women.

Finally, we meet and engage in a no-holds-barred, winner-take-all battle in front of the natives. Sheena is tall, beautiful, and very muscular. She is dressed in a tiny zebra-skin bikini. At first, the battle is closely contested. The men cheer whenever I gain the advantage; the women do the same for my opponent. Eventually, Sheena's superior strength and fighting ability allow her to take control and dominate. At one point, I am reduced to tears of frustration as I realize that defeat is inevitable and I, and all of the men, shall soon be slaves of women.

The battle ends with me on my knees begging for mercy. Sheena then encircles my neck with a leather collar to which she attaches a leash. She strips me naked and makes me kneel and kiss her feet. She then announces that this is the natural order and that all should comply. Most of the men immediately strip and sink to their knees as the women remove the collars from around their own necks and affix them to the necks of the men. The few men that resist are immediately subdued and beaten into submission. In their jubilation, many of the women rape their new slaves and/or force them to service them orally.

Sheena then leads me to her treehouse, where I am instructed as to my domestic duties and learn that my role in life is to serve my mistress's pleasure. I am kept naked at all times, and I am taught to use my tongue with great skill. I am trained to stay hard for long periods of time. I am never to have an orgasm without permission but must provide her with several every day. I am given permission to cum only rarely and if I do by accident am administered with various devices.

MASTURBATION: PURE FREEDOM!

I believe in masturbation, as I do in fantasy. There is so much to be learned from it, beginning with "Know thyself." Until we have masturbated and discovered that we share a unique compatibility with our genitals, we are cheating ourselves. There are many that believe lying to their child about sex is for their own good, pretending that sex doesn't exist—their genitals, at best, are invisible—will help the child's acceptance into society. I wish they would take a closer look, not just at the surface but at the deeper effects these lies have had on their children. Perhaps they would become more open, honest, and, yes, permissive as parents.

All by ourselves, masturbation teaches that while it's lovely to lie down with a partner, there is another course of erotic pleasure that is ours alone. Ideally, we can have both. They enhance one another, as do the fantasies that we bring to each. Masturbation says, "You are whole unto yourself." Knowing this opens doors, options, a deeper knowledge of self. It makes us stronger individuals.

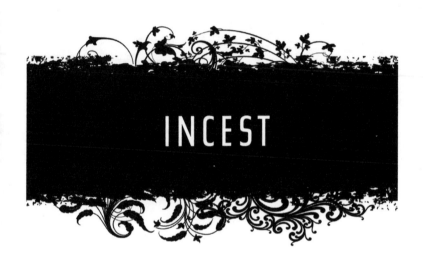

INCEST

INCEST
"All in the Family" Fantasies

Tentatively, we reach back in time for an understanding of our sexual lives. While we like to think we are architects of our sexuality, we know our past helps provide answers as to why we prefer a certain form of sex, or fear it, or have decided to altogether leave sex out of our lives. Incest is one of those acts in our culture that has always been painful to address.

Hollywood's nonexistent incest was safe, reassuring, although at some level, along with Hollywood's nonexistent homosexuality, we knew it lacked truth. I don't refer to films willing to look at the darker side of life but to satisfying blockbusters such as *Back to the Future*, where the teenage boy kisses his now-teenage mother, both instantly knowing it is wrong, a sexual turnoff. "It's like kissing my brother," she says.

We saw the look of our teenage friend's father as he steals a glance at his beautiful daughter or our teenage boyfriend's mother as she takes in her handsome son. Why should we address something that doesn't exist or, at the least, isn't permissible in any society we know of?

Dr. Laurence R. Tancredi, a prominent New York psychiatrist, in his book *Hardwired Behavior* says: "Sex between parent and child is forbidden in all cultures, as it is between brother and sister, but in ancient Egypt, brother and sister relationships were allowed in the royal family. In contrast, the incest taboo in some cultures may extend as far as to second-order cousins."

Cleopatra, killing her younger brother/husband when he tried to usurp power, hardly attests to the beauty of incest.

When asked if incest is permissible in any society today, Dr. Tancredi says, "Some assume there are secluded tribes, cut off from the world, where incest is an acceptable norm, but Margaret Mead assures that while incest may occur in every society, none have been discovered where it is acceptable."

I remember my schoolteacher telling our class that the great deterrent of incest is biology, citing how certain ancient empires collapsed because of inbreeding in the royal families.

Western European birthrates are dramatically falling as more educated young men and women focus on personal pleasure, career, success, holding off indefinitely on the devotion to the care and nurture of children. With all of our knowledge of birth control, is inbreeding really the reason for our aversion to incest or is it a more visceral understanding of its emotional impediments?

Incest happens now, or at least is talked about, at a rate I never encountered before. I am not just referring to fantasies of incest but to recaptured scenes of actually lying with Mom or Dad in the parental bed.

Memories of incest range from so nightmarish they are forced to the deepest recesses of the mind to memories as sweet as family picnics at the shore. To this day, many of these men and women with positive feelings continue their intimate relationships with members of the family or, at the very least, maintain through fantasies the erotic thrill of what was once shared.

We tend to exaggerate our parents' flaws and weaknesses. They can be projected onto us, threatening our survival. These magnified flaws help repress sexually fantasizing our parents. When a man asks in the heat of sex, "Who's your daddy?" an honest remark would often kill the moment. It certainly would in my case. In the throes of passion, who wants to hear a long speech about not having a father? Longing to submit, we respond, "You…you are, Daddy!"

But we can fantasize about other, similar people without these flaws. It's said that "girls marry their fathers; boys their mothers." I wouldn't know, but I've heard it so often, I believe there must be some truth to it. Jesse, after attending to his plus-size mother's and aunts' sore feet to much appreciation, now craves to caress the feet of heavyset women. Jesse, never a victim of incest, never imagines a family member in his fantasies.

But the flaws of our parents and older siblings are but small hurdles to sexually fantasizing about them when considering the power of these gods. In their turn, the rush they feel as they are idolized by beautiful, innocent, adoring eyes can be a powerful force. Given the right ingredients, can we resist submission to them?

In my small immediate family—my mother, my sister, and I—the ingredients weren't there. I envied my sister, Susie, for her beauty, kindness, for being everything a girl should be. My mother's constant focus on her, judging her walk, talk, attire, even with a constant critical eye, only enforced my invisibility. I'd still like to know how it feels to be so beautiful your mother can't take her eyes off of you, even if only to nag.

It forced me to go out into the world, find friendship wherever I could. Eventually, it gave me the freedom to write these books. I denied my envy with a firm belief in my superiority. After all, I, two years younger, could beat my sister at any game, get better grades, and be the most popular girl in town.

My anger, a deeply hidden rage, left no recipe for incestuous thoughts of my mother and sister. But I understand the power of incest. I know how it feels to worship the god of the family.

My grandfather was younger than most grandfathers. He made a point of this by insisting I call him Daddy Colbert instead of Granddaddy. Unlike my shy, nervous mother, Daddy Colbert enjoyed strength, power, money, sex. When he entered a room, people took notice. I adored Daddy Colbert. I wanted to be him.

During his brief visits, I'd run and jump on his lap. He'd laugh with approval as Susie disappeared into the wallpaper and Mother anxiously attended to his requests. My true prize of getting straight As, winning competitions, selling the most rat poison door to door was seeing his face light up with a loving look of approbation, to know that I was Daddy Colbert's girl.

After leaving the South to go North in my first year of college, I finally acquired the fine curve of an ass, a face men didn't seem to mind. Suddenly, my 5'10" body and grade average weren't handicaps. My looks came too late to ever fully trust, compliments always seeming directed to someone behind me. But I remember the wonderful thrill when Daddy Colbert would now come to New York on business and show me off to his friends: "Gentlemen, this is my granddaughter!"

Once, while having drinks with him at his hotel, the evening ended with an invitation to join him in his suite. I declined as prettily as possible, hugged him, and hailed a taxi.

At nineteen, having experienced every sexual pleasure except penetration, I was still a technical virgin. Had my first technically nonvirginal act been with my grandfather, the one person I had always been in awe of, how could anyone else ever compare? How impossible would it be for me to let go, for us to return to the relationship that I cherished?

Some people who have had incestuous relationships with parents they worship can only orgasm by fantasizing about that parent, no matter who the lover is. Had I joined my grandfather in his suite, would that now be me?

THE SINGLE PARENT
"What a Big Bed for One Person"

In single-parent families, there is no fear of punishment from the other parent when the child desires the mother or father. Amelie remembers on Sunday lying in the big bed next to her father, while her mother was downstairs making pancakes. "He would be turned away from me, reading the paper, and I would be lying next to his back, running my fingers up and down its expanse. But I would always remember—perhaps glad and fearful—that Mom was down in the kitchen, and she could come up at any time." Young Amelie had a sense of danger and excitement but also knew the boundary and the rules.

When there is a second parent, the child may not have the incest fantasy because of fear of reprisals from the other parent. Such fantasies are repressed or put out of consciousness. With no fear of retribution when the child crawls into the bed of a single parent, it is the parent's responsibility to deal with the child's awakening sexuality. How we deal with the natural processes of the little boy wanting to sleep with mommy, the little girl's naked dance for daddy will affect their entire lives. Pushing the child away with disgust can be as harmful as acting on the advances.

Often, it's the single, lonely parent who has plenty of room in a large, cold bed. Men and women alike recount growing up in bed with either Mom or Dad. If this modern sharing of the big bed has been consistent since earliest childhood, it's understandable that sons and daughters will think nothing of the arrangement when it comes to their turn at parenting.

The child who grows up in a parent's bed feels he or she belongs to that parent. It's difficult enough for young people to separate from mother and father, who, without sex, already have an extraordinary hold over us. If we grew up in the parental bed, how will traditional monogamy not be boring?

Young children can be seductive, but he or she who keeps a roof over the family and provides sustenance has all the power in the world in these young eyes. Playing in the big bed, pillow fighting, is one thing, but sleeping beside Mom and/or Dad night after night, these first tentative, innocent arousals can be knitted into the erotic imagination. How can they not?

Does a single parent whose own life is barren of sex bring a different attitude to a child's sexual curiosity? What do the children know of a parent's loneliness, the emptiness in his or her bed at night? When a child sees a parent cry, it is confusing and frightening; after all, this is the person upon whom life depends, and crying is a sign of weakness, frailty, arousing not just sympathy in a child but anxiety.

To children, the parent is god, source of everything they need. The idea that this colossus's needs might go beyond their world doesn't occur. They have everything; they have us, and they control our lives. "But, Mommy, I'm here," the boy says when she weeps. Should she answer "But, darling, you're not enough," his heart sinks.

As for my friend, needing me to powder him, baby him, eternally craving to be adored, his incest fantasy was practically carved in stone.

Sylvia

Sylvia, a young widow poised to marry her late husband's brother, is waiting until their wedding night to make love. How will her loneliness for her late husband, manifesting into sexual fantasies of her son, affect all their lives?

It was several months since Sam died when my son, Freddy, who's now eleven, came to my bed in the middle of the night asking if he could stay with me a while. He'd had a nightmare about his dad and was crying. I welcomed him into my bed, and he put his head on my breast. I comforted him and stroked his hair. We drifted off to sleep. The next morning, I felt really good. Freddy tells me that I must have been tired because Sam Junior woke up, and so he brought him to bed so I could nurse him. I am a really sound sleeper. Freddy thought I was awake because I opened my gown for Junior to nurse. Freddy tells me that he took Junior back to the baby bed because he knew I didn't want him to get used to sleeping with me—especially since now I would be marrying his uncle Kenneth.

I'm a good mother. I love my boys and would never sexually abuse them. I always want them to know that they can trust me, that I'd only act in their best interest. But I've had this erotic dream, which I admit, I've also used for masturbation. The orgasms it brings on are like explosions. I think it may be my way to mix reality and fantasy, to bring Sam back, as Freddy looks so much like his father.

In the fantasy, I'm just lying there when Freddy climbs into bed. He snuggles up to my breasts and starts to lick my nipples like a baby seeking his mother's milk. He gently takes my hand and puts it on his erect penis. I concentrate on pretending I'm asleep, but I am aroused when I feel that he has pushed his underwear down, and he is almost the size of his dad. He starts talking like Sam: "Oh, Sylvie, I love you. Come on, honey, give it to Daddy." By this time, I am so aroused I decide to pretend I'm having an erotic dream and start begging, saying, "Baby, don't leave. Make love to me. Fuck me. Fuck me, damn it!" Needless to say, Freddy is obedient and fucks me but then pulls out before he cums, then leaves before I "wake up."

Reading this, I wonder how Sylvia will accept other women in her son's life if he continues to be the focus of her sexual fantasy? Should he marry, is she doomed to become the interfering mother-in-law, only wanting the best for her son, a role no other woman can fulfill, or because of her guilt, believing she's a bad mother, will she overcompensate by showing little judgment of any of his sexual partners?

I understand loneliness, I have been there, but the harm done in incest is not readily discernible. Being allowed into the Queen/King's bed feels like an honor. If it is mother, the breast, once the child's favorite cushion, is absolute heaven.

Without another grown-up upon whom to lean, single parents often do not, or cannot, hide from their children their loneliness, tension, fear, the lexicon of emotion that might more appropriately be shared by a partner. No matter how we cover, at some level, children know the truth.

I'm pro-fantasy, as escape, leading us into a higher realm of ecstasy. But children are intuitive, sensing if they are in the parent's bed to be comforted from their nightmare or if for another reason. The child we bathe, protect, and feed is recording life's lessons, not irrefutable, but still, they will be the bedrock from which will emerge the erotic circuitry wired into a complex adult. Hopefully, Sylvia's second husband, her husband's brother—keeping it all in the family—will fill the emotional vacuum from her husband's death.

I've always imagined how my own life would be different had there been a man in the house. I like to think he would not have been as occupied with cleanliness as my dear mother, something I've inherited. But I've never doubted that my own fondness for breaking the rules came from a very early determination *not* to be like her. I could never imagine my mother discussing with anyone a "daddy fantasy." Mine are not a daddy I've known and touched but, like Daddy Colbert, the all-powerful loving male that will force me gently into submission, into ecstasy.

Kieran

Kieran, an attractive twenty-one-year-old working as a "go-go boy," speaks lightheartedly, reminding me of my own story of the missing father. We fantasize not of the father we know but of the father about whom we dream.

My mother was married to someone else when she got pregnant by my father. Yeah, that marriage didn't work out. She pretty much raised me on my own. I think she always knew I was gay. Like she says, "How many little boys pluck their eyebrows?"

The whole incest thing wasn't an issue. I only saw my father a few times a year. But now he's in the Army, and about a year ago, he told me he's bisexual. Suddenly, he's all about how beautiful I am and coming on to me but not like totally explicit. I told him, "You gotta cut out that shit. It ain't happening. I'll cut your dick off if you ever try to fuck me with it." His attitude's been a lot better since then.

Maybe it's 'cause I didn't see my dad much growing up, and I'm not into my dad at all, but I have a big daddy fantasy. I won't see a guy under twenty-five unless he's super mature and, of course, hot. I had one boyfriend in his forties who's a porn star. I met him online, he started calling me his "Baby," and I called him "Daddy." When we met, it was so fucking hot. I got hard the second he said in my ear: "Is Baby gonna make Daddy happy? You gonna be a good boy?" Was I ever! It was amazing sex for a few months. He'd touch me, and I'd quiver. Then, he got all crazy because he found out I slept with a few other guys. I couldn't believe it. What did he think I was doing when he was on a film shoot, baking cookies? Jesus, he's a porn star!

I find it telling that one of the beliefs held up by the patriarchal society, well into the feminist years, was that "real men" didn't suffer from early sexual abuse. Not that long ago, no one explored or wrote about the fact that some men, as boys, were molested. The abused man himself simply did not want to admit to something as "unmanly" as carrying those demeaning scars. As women joined in the stature of "provider," men could more easily own up to their vulnerabilities.

We women, now the head of most single-parent families, have become more assertive with regard to incest. Without the presence of an adult male, more women have access to the authority that comes with economic independence. When a woman takes a son to her bed these days, or an aunt her nephew, as in Case's situation, I suppose the act is less fraught with anxiety. We are still taught that the man is the aggressor, that he unequivocally desires sex. But what effect does this have on the boy's life?

Case

I'm in my fifties now but first had sex with an older, somewhat domineering aunt when I was fourteen. I never shared this with anyone until I went online and read about others who've had similar family experiences. I've written a few people on Craigslist and was glad to know that it occurs more than I thought.

My aunt's still alive, but we rarely see each other except at family funerals. She's somewhat the matriarch and something tells me I wasn't the only young man in the family she's had relations with. I was sent to her one summer to help out around her bed and breakfast. It was around the time when I learned how to masturbate and ejaculate. I'd used my mother's and older sister's panties to wrap around my penis and masturbate because it felt so good.

I started doing this with my aunt's half-slips the first week I was there, and she walked in on me in the bathroom while I was doing it. She screamed at me, and I started to freak out and was crying when she pulled me close to her and told me it was okay, she wouldn't tell anyone. But I had to do exactly as she instructed; otherwise, there would be real problems in the family.

She had me run a bath, then she stepped out of her clothes and into the tub where I was told to scrub her back and everywhere. I was more scared than turned on, but after she was done, I helped towel her off, and she had me strip and get into the tub where I cleaned myself in her bath water.

She kept having me soap my penis until it was hard and then she hosed me off, and we went into her bedroom, where she proceeded to teach me how to pleasure her, with my hands, my mouth, and, eventually, with my penis. She had had a hysterectomy, so I learned it was safe to ejaculate in or around her, and we had sex almost daily for the entire summer. We would sleep together in her bed, and I remember many Sunday mornings waking up and having her straddle my face until she was ready for intercourse.

I now masturbate regularly to mature/young websites that show pictures of middle-aged women and young men having sex. Being in my fifties, mature may be younger than I am!

When my wife and I were more sexually active, we'd tell each other stories about past sexual experiences and even role-played some of the scenarios. She thought the most outrageous thing either of us had done was when she had sex in front of an open hotel window with a past lover. I never told her about that summer at my aunt's, but it's embossed in my brain.

I find that some women who have been with underaged boys feel they are actually doing a service, teaching them the skills of satisfying a woman. Other women may be aware that sex with the boy is for their own sexual pleasure, but they feel the boy couldn't perform if it weren't consensual. Their justification gives them little concern for the long-term effects.

Before feminism, if a man did confess to having been molested as a child, there was reluctance to give credence or sympathy. With a woman, we understood, sympathized with her alcoholism, bitchery, insomnia. But men were expected to "take it like a man!" What kind of fantasies were created, how were they acted out for these men? How are they acted out now for people, still reluctant to show weakness and vulnerability, who are unable to deal with their abuse in a healthy manner?

IMPRINTS OF INCEST
"Unforgettable, That's What You Are"

Women's absence from their children's lives, due to career and work, isn't the only reason younger contributors to this book have experienced so much more sex than the generations before them. There is also the biggest educator of all, one that doesn't discriminate—the media. Studies have shown children who spend more time in front of the TV and computer from an early age experience sex earlier.

We live in unique times. We have a yen for a certain kind of sex, sit at our computers where, sure enough, someone else has been there, done that, and is perhaps still living it. There is no precedent for the thought process aided by the Internet today. The plethora of incest sites go from parent/child/siblings all the way up to and beyond quintuplets and their family pets. The Internet's long arm, with its endless supply confirming the popularity of these sexual fantasies, has a way of eliminating almost any nagging sense of responsibility.

The parental bed has always been the sought-after terrain that children wanted to own. Now, in a cyber world, there is a quick stop to a site confirming, even prompting, parents to invite the child to climb aboard, to tuck in beside Mom or Dad.

Books have been written about the "beauty" of incest. Whether there can be positive aspects, in all my years, I've never heard of anyone resentful because they *weren't* molested as a child.

The "polarization" of a young person's life that goes on when a parent involves a child in a sexual act isn't far from the kind of isolation that occurs when young people "lose themselves" in cyberspace addictions. In the end, sex with Mom or Dad can eliminate the meaningful experience of sexual awakening with people of one's own choice.

In the days of my earlier books, women would be so cautious about admitting to erotic imaginings, they would often have the entire fantasy in places such as a steam bath, where the swirling clouds of steam hid her face as well as the identity of the person approaching her as she lay naked, awaiting her invented assignation. The Internet is the new "facelessness," the anonymity engaging us into the raw sex we desire without societal reprimand.

Many fantasies of incest began as a reality long ago. When we are young in the parental bed, what do we know of the dark side of incest? Having been invited to share the bed of the King and/or Queen, the most powerful people in our lives, what later invitations can measure up? Twenty, thirty years later, our imagination still trips back to what seemed like paradise.

Sex is a powerful tie. It arouses the need and desire to bond and merge with the partner who has brought these feelings. Should every sexual partner later in life be compared with Mom or Dad, the first all-powerful caretakers? I'm not speaking of the pyrotechnics of sex but the deep emotional feelings that are aroused by intercourse. We will never have with another person the unique emotional attachment that we had with our parents nor should we expect others to provide it. The purpose or business within a family focuses on the child's growing up and away from the parents and into his or her own identity.

Sex is usually the act of separation, orgasm being a climax that confirms in the most pleasurable way our existence, unique unto ourselves. Jodi says that when she first had sexual intercourse with her boyfriend on the couch in her parents' den, each time they "did it," she felt that she had broken away, "naturally," from her parents and her childhood. To mix up, to confuse that brilliant statement of individuation with parental/child symbiosis, can forever confuse the child's future. Too pliable and needy, the soft clay may bear the imprint of your body parts for the rest of your child's life.

For Lorena and Erica, the images are transfixed. How can they let go, erase them and start their journey afresh, on equal grounds with a loving partner?

Lorena

Raised in a strict Baptist household, Lorena says she was about five years old when she began to masturbate.

My first sexual experience was with my father. I was about seven when my dad asked me in a hushed way if I would "jack him off." I didn't know what it meant, but I could tell by his tone that it was naughty.

He would have me lubricate his dick with an oil and masturbate him while he held my naked body next to his with one arm. He usually held a pornographic magazine in the other arm. I remember my arm would get tired, and I would have to switch.

Sometimes, he would have me lay on my back while he looked at my pussy and kissed it. One time, he had me take a shower with him, and we washed each other. I dreaded being home alone with him, but I was ashamed to tell anyone. He always gave me money afterward and told me not to tell. This went on until I reached puberty.

I got pregnant and secretly had an abortion when I was eighteen. Sex with boys was disappointing. I masturbate almost every day. In my fantasies, a man, or men, whom I do not know forces me into various sex acts. I am either physically overpowered or coerced through the threat of violence. Violence itself turns me off. As a second job, I was secretly a call girl for about a year. I made excellent money, but I wouldn't recommend it for everyone.

Erica

I was sexually abused and regularly penetrated by my oldest brother, starting when I was about twelve years old. There was no one to tell, as I had a stepmother. My grandfather was also sexually inappropriate with me. He never penetrated me or took my clothes off, but it was sexual abuse. He kissed me, forcing his tongue into my mouth and pressing me against him so I would feel his erection. I found my first husband couldn't sexually satisfy me, and I became sexually active with other men. After we divorced, I was raped by the first man I went out with, became pregnant, and had an abortion. I could not handle children as a single parent.

My fantasies have always bothered me a little. I can only guess it is because of the sexual abuse. But I have always been very stimulated by taboo situations—parent and child, interracial, same-sex lovemaking, clergy and parishioner, older and younger. I think I want to share the discomfort of potentially abusive fantasies as a person who has been abused.

I have a fantasy of a daughter and father having sex while Mom is away. The thrill of the risk of discovery is an additional pleasure. Mom makes a phone call home to see how things are going while she is out of town. The daughter tells Mom, while she and Dad are having sex, that Dad cannot come to the phone, as his mouth is full or he is working hard on the pump. The daughter and mother have a long conversation about other things while the sex goes on. It is more stimulating to both of them knowing the mother might be able to hear some noise but will not suspect what is causing it.

INCEST FANTASIES OF WISH FULFILLMENT, OR,
"Love Thy Parents, More Than They Know"

One of the positive values of fantasy is that it allows us to play out desires we know we cannot fulfill in real life without hurting ourselves and others, such as sleeping with a best friend's spouse. The same could be said of incestuous thoughts of one's family members. If the thoughts are there, if they arouse you, so be it. Putting these fantasies into action is *altogether different and irreversible.*

Is the surrender to incest the cry for intimacy of a sort that was totally missing in the first years of life? Do family members turn to one another for missing parental/maternal intimacy? When there's only a mother and a son in the house, does the emptiness cry out for everyone to sleep in one bed?

Disturbing as the intrafamily sexual fantasies can be, I sometimes hear these voices crying out for not so much sex but the kind of familial intimacy that used to define us, a tight, loyal group of Mom, Dad, and children.

Leigh sees her fantasies with her uncle as a way of repairing and rewriting the sad reality of her childhood. "I never got along with my family, and these erotic fantasies with my uncle could be a desire for that harmonious family relationship. In any case, if I could make this fantasy happen, I'd leap at the chance."

Leigh

I am thirty-six years old, and my sex life with my husband is pathetic. If it weren't for the kids, I'd be gone in a minute. He only cares about his own satisfaction in bed, and I've come to realize, after all this time, it's not going to change. I've given it my best shot but now realize it's hopeless. In the early days, I believed that I turned him on so much that he couldn't control himself; now I know he just uses me to get his rocks off. I've done everything for him that any man could want (I mean everything!), but he won't spend any amount of time pleasuring me. Fantasy and masturbation are much more satisfying to me than sex with this clod. I dream of being with a man who will make love to me for hours—someone who wants to do more in bed than fuck for twenty seconds and then go to sleep. I think about men I know as well as strangers (a highway patrolman who stops me for speeding and ends up eating me on the hood of my car). When I fantasize about guys that I know, it's usually a very passionate and sensual scene with lots of kissing, touching, massaging, licking, sucking, and talking (as well as fucking).

As I masturbate, sometimes my fantasy wanders off into other areas—being with another woman, group sex, incest, rape.

I started masturbating when I was five. One time, I started wiggling when I was alone with a neighbor man. In no time at all, he was on the floor next to me, with his hand under me, encouraging me to keep wiggling on top of his hand. When he found out what a horny little kid I was, he progressed to putting his hand in my pants (that was easy, since he already knew how much I liked having my pussy rubbed), licking my pussy, finger-fucking me (he let me watch in the mirror), showing me his penis (seeing it become erect was my biggest fascination)—and finally, at my urging ("just stick it in"), penetrating me and ejaculating inside me.

By the time I was twelve years old, I also had been fondled by a teacher during a private lesson, ravished by my swimming coach, and gang-raped by a bunch of teenage boys in their summer fort. (I loved every minute of each of these encounters and started looking for opportunities to get laid.) I also sucked the tits of an older teenage girlfriend. Besides fondling and sucking each other's tits, we kissed and rubbed our pussies together and felt each other up. I can't explain it. I just love sex. Always have.

My fantasy is inspired. I am twelve years old and staying with my uncle at his ranch for a weekend. He tells me I need a nice hot bath after horseback riding. I fantasize that we've always been close, have spent a lot of time together, and we know and love each other very much. I trust him so much that I would let him do anything to me—and he knows it. He takes my hand and helps me in the bath. He immerses my body in the warm, soothing water as he adores the sight of my naked body—mature enough to have small firm breasts but young enough to be without pubic hair. He joins me in the tub. His soft penis and scrotum hang way down as he climbs in and sits down next to me and pulls me onto his lap. He talks quietly. Then, his hand slides down my flat belly to my soft, smooth pussy, and he sticks his middle finger in my slit and feels me up for a long time.

He says he knows another way to make my pussy feel good, and he leads me out of the tub and lays me down on his warm water bed. With my legs together, he rubs my vulva and presses on the mound over my pubic in a circular motion. His finger probes deeper into my pussy, searching to see if I am getting wet. I try to open my legs, but he holds them together. He brings his face to my pussy. He licks me from asshole to belly button, over and over. After a while, his cock is aching for some attention, and he tells me how to suck him. He pulls out and squeezes his shaft to delay his ejaculation and whispers in my ear that he needs to put his cock in my pussy now.

He has a look of pure delight on his face as he watches his cock slide in and out of my little hairless pussy. After a while, he starts shoving it in a little harder and occasionally looks up to see my small round tits dance as he plunges into me. He cries out in pleasure as he fucks my tight virgin cunt.

Beverly

I'm in my twenties now, and I never felt guilty masturbating to fantasies, but my fantasies have never been based on love. My most recurrent fantasy concerns my father. I would hate to have sex with my father, but I suppose it turns me on just because it's wrong. I'm almost positive it hasn't entered my dad's head. He would be disgusted. I hope I don't offend anyone.

My mother has gone away for the weekend, for some reason, and I am watching TV with my father. The film contains some explicit sexual scene. I start getting hot and gradually start to masturbate. My dad ignores this. Soon, my father wonks off, as I do. I suggest we might as well fuck each other. My father is hesitant, as he is a conventional man. When I kneel before him and reach for his huge beautiful cock, I tell him how much I want to fuck the cock that made me. My father becomes wild, ripping off my skirt and bra. My tits tumble out to meet my father's fingers, which caress and circle my erect nipples. My father now laps away at my clitoris, ecstatic at his new experience, while I finger-fuck my sopping-wet cunt until I have a heart-stopping orgasm. I get up to see my father's reaction. He tells me what a big girl I am, and he carries me upstairs and gives me a bath. Then, we head off to Mom and Dad's room for a night of endless fucking in every conceivable position.

My dad buys a separate apartment for our sex sessions near to my home, and we pursue a secret affair. The room always smells of sex, for we are there at every opportunity.

Tilda

I'm a mother of three teenage children and have been married for over thirty years. I feel so awful having all these feelings and having fantasies and experiences like I do. My husband is loving and caring, and our sex is just as good as when we first got married. I am faithful and dutiful and very happy.

I have fantasies, however; the power of the mind to be immensely erotic does not die with age. I masturbate having such thoughts, both with my husband and when I am alone. I fantasize about sex with my father, who I dearly loved. Nothing like I imagine ever happened—I was never sexually abused; our family was warm and close and loving. So, this is not some deeply repressed memory. This is just a fantasy.

I always have fantasized about him for as long as I can recall. It confuses me, excites me, thrills me, scares me even. I do not understand it. When I was three or four, I accidentally touched my father's penis. He was taking a shower, and I, as usual, was sitting in the bathroom talking to him. He got out of the shower, and I do not know why, but I reached out and touched his penis. I began to stroke it in my hand, and I remember now, clear as day, that it began to grow and grow, until it was hard and darkish purple. My father took my hand away firmly and told me I shouldn't have done that.

In my fantasy, I am fifteen years old, and my father is forty-five. In real life, he was a large, handsome, muscular man, a laborer/builder, with a thick head of black hair that never really thinned as he grew older. In the fantasy, I am in the house alone when he comes up behind me, presses himself against me, placing his large yet gentle hands over my breasts. Then, he carries me upstairs, I know what for.

Deirdre

Deirdre is a black woman in her thirties living in a large metropolitan area.

This is the fantasy that I had when I first experienced the joy of an orgasm during intercourse: It starts with my birth. When the doctor told my father that it was a girl, he takes me and kisses me on my pussy, and he has kissed it every day since. (It's never my father's face in the fantasy.) At the age of five, he started to eat my pussy, and at the age of ten, he began to finger-fuck me. He said it was to get it ready because at thirteen, he would fuck me for the first time. One day, my dad is eating my pussy and finger-fucking me, and I start sucking his prick. He's so turned on by my sucking him off. And I am so hot by his tongue and fingers that I need something bigger in me. So, I hop on top of him and *fuck him like he has never been fucked before. I am riding him really hard, and he begins to scream that this is his pussy, and he will* never let me leave him.

BROTHERLY LOVE
"The Family That Plays Together, Stays Together"

At the time of writing *My Secret Garden*, I felt unqualified to give an opinion of incest. I still try to take a nonjudgmental stance on sexual fantasy and always politely hold the doors open for consensual adults. But since my research in the early '70s, I've have a clearer understanding of the pitfalls of incest. The laws protect the child, just as we are protected from murderers and thieves.

In everything I've written, I seem to include reference to the issues of attachment and separation, these stages in life that prepare us early on for our journey as individuals. Since my writing in the early '70s, I've come to believe that when we are very young, the bedrock should be laid for our ability to believe in ourselves, alone and separate from the people who bore and raised us. It is this human brickwork, bit by bit, that allows us to strike out on our own, impatient to further the adventure of who we are.

This is the great theme of immortal stories read to small children who take them in and remember them for the rest of their lives, telling them to their own children along the way. Would Cinderella have been happier finding out that the prince is not only the best sex she's ever had but also her long-lost brother?

Slaying the dragon stands for the excruciating aloneness of separating, making it on our own. Reread Grimm, replacing the dragon with your competitive, unscrupulous new boss, "substituting" the forest primeval with the streets of the new city where you have been assigned. Sexual discovery of a new lover's body, the mirroring image of ourselves in new eyes, the reflection of ourselves is now that of an adult. A new identity we'd never have discovered had we not become a pioneer.

What a glorious discovery about oneself, falling in love, winning the man/woman of our dreams. What a great jolt of excitement when someone decides to give themselves to us, says they have seen something in us that is pure re-enforcement of selfhood. Winning someone's love in the family, well, so you beat out your brother or sister. Big deal.

Once upon a time, the close tie between parent and child was all important for the procreation and growth, the sustenance the child needed and the parent offered. But that sustenance is supposed to raise a young person to take the first steps out into the world. If the feast in the parental bed is kept available, why should the son/daughter venture forth?

A fifty-year-old woman's brother introduced her to sex when she was nine years old; then her father took over. She doesn't sound the least unhappy about the past and has absolutely no remorse for what her father did to her. In fact, she looks forward to having sex with her eighty-year-old father-in-law as a birthday present.

Another woman speaks of having sex with her sister since they were children. "Who can you trust but your sister?" she adds. Though her sister is married, they still "steal" sex together. She fantasizes finding a man to marry who would be compatible sexually with her and her sister and brother-in-law.

Men and women who have shared an incestuous relationship with a parent are sometimes evangelical about the experience. Do we proclaim the joys of what happened as an effort to camouflage ambivalence? Does having been there, in Mom or Dad's bed, feel better, more justified, if others we know have tried it too?

Sleeping alone, in one's bed, is how life on one's own begins. We learn to deal with bad dreams not by crawling closer to a parent but by understanding fear of the dark, fear of being alone, all the fears a child can only resolve by his or her own self, not cuddled against the parental body. I believe the more nonthreatening the path of incest becomes, the more we're stepping back over the millenniums into tribal times or even further back to when we lived as a pack. This is my own personal belief.

During pillow talk, a boyfriend once asked me, "So, who was your first?" I replied, "I don't remember." "Bullshit," he said. "Everybody remembers their first time." I said, "Really? I think people remember their best times. I had so many firsts, I wouldn't know where to start. Do you count the first peck on the cheek?" He said, "Who's the first guy who fucked you?" He was right. The memory of that first time is so vivid, it's hard to believe it happened such a time long ago.

The act of sex, the leading up to it, going through it with someone, can be one of the great steps into one's new, individuated life. This crucial business of separation, the delicate balance way back when we are too young to control what happens, is the foundation that we will live with for the rest of our lives. Symbiotic oneness in the first year, the loving gaze, the adoration, then separating frees us to be our own person without forever reaching for that missing love.

If the move beyond home is complicated by intimate ties to Mom, Dad, siblings, we are going to be less inclined to open doors, to take risks, to forge friendships and love relationships with the people we meet.

Sex isn't just pleasure. In choosing the people we want to lie down with, we are betting on ourselves. When it works, when sex with a new person opens us to one another in that rare way, it is one of the great gifts.

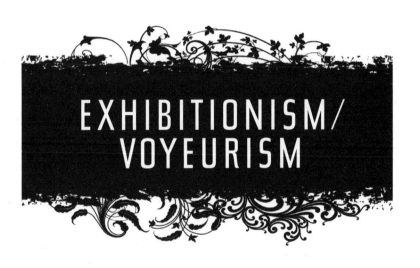

EXHIBITIONISM/
VOYEURISM

EXHIBITIONISM/VOYEURISM

I remember glancing up from the bed where I lay with my lover to see a man standing in the doorway, smoking a cigarette, watching us. We were at a guesthouse in Martinique. There was a moment when the stranger's eyes met mine. I felt no fear or disapproval, perhaps because the guesthouse was small and intimate. If I'd cried out, I'd have awakened other guests, or was my silence part of my own exhibitionism, which was in turn part of coming of age and accepting who I was?

I'd chosen to be with this interesting man beside me in bed, knowing he was on a personal voyage of sexual discovery. I was crazy about him, a brilliant intellectual, a voyeur, and an exhibitionist. These were the wild and crazy '70s when we were beginning to throw off our chains and stretch our libidos. The music, the dance, the costumes that we wore were all part of this age of discovery. We who wanted to be seen now didn't have to hide it. This was central not just to the costumes but to what we wrote, how we danced and spoke. It was the beginning of in vogue exhibitionism, for both men and women.

Perhaps the entire country didn't instantly jump on board, but New York City and other urban centers were a voyeur's smorgasbord. It was impossible *not* to take in the man approaching, his "package" so adroitly arranged in his tight crotch you could see the outline of every twist and turn of his penis. The competition for the eye was over the top! "Take me in! Feast your eyes! Look at me, for I am hungry to be seen!" We were both patrons and artists in this new sexual catwalk.

With every door my lover opened, I followed, until one night, the door he opened was the beginning of our end. We were at a wild party, and in the bedroom he entered were three people embroiled in a scene straight out of his favorite fantasy. He stood at the foot of the bed, transfixed. So, there we were, the woman watching her man watching the three people in bed. I wanted my lover to turn and see me. I might as well have asked a famished dog not to sniff at a sizzling steak. His eyes full, he stripped and fed his starved erotic soul, no exaggeration. It was absolutely in keeping with who he was. I bowed out. Had he been just a friend and not my lover, I'd have joined in. But I was learning my limits.

Designers today still try to recapture the excitement of the '60s and '70s when fashion was caught up in a sexual revolution. Of course, it's not about the clothes and music. It's us. In revolutionizing the configuration of how men and women are. As we remove more and more "Do Nots," there are less rules to bend or break. There is less differentiation between man and woman. As the sexes become more interchangeable, there is less spark. For sex to come alive, there has to be a me and a you, a space between us for the spark of eros to jump and ignite. There may be a lot more sex but perhaps without as much fire. Instead of patrons and artists of this new sexual catwalk, we become the blasé gatekeepers. With more strutting and less looking, the exhibitionist in us goes hungry.

Ours is a shaky world these days. It is easy to get lost in it, so crowded are the streets, so intense the competition to be recognized. There is little left to shock, few new dishes left for our eyes to devour. Everything and everyone has been taken to the extreme. Where does the exhibitionist in us go from here?

Feeling invisible in a crowded world of anxious, competitive, angry people is a dynamite position with a hair trigger. When it comes to sex, these feelings don't dissipate. The rising fever to orgasm is a furnace that draws on all available fuel.

How "natural" that we reach in fantasies for the sensations that have been hounding us all day. This time, we make them work for us. All day long, we've felt "unseen, unimportant, invisible." We spread our legs, making "them" see our most private parts or we imagine we are voyeurs of others' most intimate moments. Without having to do anything, not having to work or strive or even seduce, we feed our eyes, which feed our soul, and feel whole again.

Is it so surprising today that fantasies of exhibitionism and voyeurism are one of the most prevalent themes? Craigslist ads like these have become common, ordinary.

Show off in public

Looking to show off in public spot or in a restroom. Would love to let you get a nice look and maybe even more if it's hot. Please email back with a location and we will make it work. Want to let you see it all!

Daddy's little girl likes showing off

I'm pretty, white, 22, 5´5˝, thin, blonde and looking to strip for an older guy, have him watch me parade in sexy panties. You'll possibly get to watch me masturbate. This is not for sex. There will be no body contact. You just get to watch.

Daddy Seeking Skinny Skater Type

Are you a hot skinny skater type in your 20's? How about hanging out, having a few beers, you strip off your shirt to show off your tight smooth skinny chest for me to worship and adore? I'm 45, very in shape, gwm 5´10 165 shaved head, great chest, hot nipples, fun, intelligent and very imaginative. Let's see how we could meet each others needs.

Whether in fantasy or reality, voyeurs/exhibitionists capture and hold the people they are watching or demand that others look at them. Either way, the theme is one of substantiality, solidity, reality, and domination.

EXHIBITIONISM, OR,
"Don't Turn That Dial!"

Today, the competition for the eye is intense. Never in modern times has there been so much public display of body parts. What makes the competition more intense is that both men and women want to be seen.

With more single parents and both parents working, it follows that fewer infants receive as much of mother's gaze that first critical year. Being seen by mother, gazed at, is necessary for us to let go, secure in mother's love. Without mother's gaze, we will always search for it, never totally separated into our own individual person. Should we really be surprised when the super-wealthy, raised by nannies and au pairs, end up on YouTube sex videos?

It is hard to prove that more children are receiving less of mother's gaze, but from the increase I've seen in men's and women's fantasies of exhibitionism, I believe it's probable. Are Paris Hilton and Britney Spears so scantily attired because they can't afford more clothes? Is Justin Timberlake really bringing sexy back or saying, "Please look at me!"? Would any young man today be embarrassed to discover that his pants are hanging below his underwear? As The Bachelor parades nearly naked for the twenty-five expectant, revealingly dressed young women competing for him, the standard of dress becomes increasingly eroticized, the competition heating up.

We were, in fact, raised not to stare. It doesn't matter whether our reaction to the exhibitionist is a smile of pleasure or shock. It's almost as though they aren't really sure until we see them that they matter.

In the past, certainly, women dressed up to be seen, admired, and chosen. But there was a dance to it: women weren't supposed to be aware of the exhibition, and men weren't supposed to stare in an obvious way, as in, "Why, his eyes practically undressed me!"

It was quite a charade: women would spend hours and all their money on "looking good," but when a compliment came their way, a typical response was, "Oh, this old thing?"

Young children feed on getting attention by running naked through the house. It's a game but not "just" a game. Every time we look and exclaim, the child feels more substantial. And it's not just the act of getting oneself seen that excites. There is a sense of power in "grabbing" someone's gaze, taking their attention away from whatever else it was on. The trick is to hold the eye, capture it, and, in essence, dominate with one's exhibitionism or voyeurism.

With less "domination" within the home, wherein parents ensured their children's corporeality by making them feel "watched," as in taken care of, children feel more invisible. The small child doesn't say, "No, don't look at me!" to his mother. The youngster looks over his shoulder to be sure mother's eye is, indeed, on him. It is only with time and a sense of identity that the child begins to seek privacy and venture farther away from home so as to exercise this growing sense of corporeal self.

With both men and women more into exhibitionism—looking good, being seen, drawing attention to themselves be it ever so discreet or not, the competition for the passing gaze has heated up. Spending on plastic surgery, cosmetics, fashion are at all-time highs. Beauty, owning it, using it in this age of equality, continues at a faster rate. As my attractive thirty-four-year-old gay friend, Saul, proudly says, referring to his wealthy fifty-two-year-old partner of six years: "I'm his trophy wife, thanks to the gifts God has bestowed on me: the nose job, da Vinci veneers, hair plugs, and the gym pass. I'm told they bring out my natural beauty."

MALE FANTASIES OF EXHIBITIONISM, OR,
"Thanks for Noticing My Zipper's Undone"

Before the sexual revolution, we were told in innumerable ways, from psychoanalysts and psychiatrists to books, movies, friends, and family, that men were the voyeurs, women the exhibitionists. Imagine, all those years we were boxed into these narrow definitions of what it was to be male or female.

One of the healthiest offshoots of feminism is that today men have returned to the mirror, to looking good, wanting to be seen and admired. Not only can men enjoy getting themselves looked at and admired, but women can now "feast their eyes." I am thinking of the great explosion of color alone in men's clothing—pink and powder blue ties, fuchsia shirts, bright yellow, the rainbow.

When I think about the old days, I wonder how my male friends, who love to dress and be admired, stood it. It was scandalous when Elvis gyrated his hips, but one could say he did it for fortune and fame. The average man on the street fed his exhibitionistic needs by being king of the home, adored by wife and children. He could not dress to be seen without eliciting question to his sanity and, even worse, his heterosexuality.

A psychoanalyst recently mentioned treating former monks who had left the church. "After hiding themselves for years, these men had the most violent, burning fantasies of exhibitionism, even after they married." Should the church be better equipped to handle these men's needs? I'm not suggesting allowing the monks to occasionally streak, but for some, it seems unhealthy to ignore the great natural desire/need to be seen. Perhaps that is why, on occasions, it is known that some monks have resorted to Peter's method below.

Peter

I'm a thirty-six-year-old married man, and my fantasies and facts have merged in my life. My fantasies are, in fact, just a short extension of reality because I am a confirmed exhibitionist, unbeknownst to my wife. I have spent years since my teens manufacturing situations in which I expose myself to women but not in the "classic" sense of wrenching open a grubby raincoat to flash my prick at some innocent passing victim. I dress up in ways that allow me to give the impression *that I am unwittingly giving an unexpected view of my genitals. I once wore a pair of jogging shorts adapted to my exhibitionism. I cut out the crotch so that when I sat down, I could flop out my genitals. Also, I have cut a circle of cloth from the backside of the trousers, which leaves my bum exposed.*

Today, sometimes I think, if there is a voyeur out there who is happy with his or her lot and not wishing he were an exhibitionist instead, he or she must be in paradise. Underwear is no longer required. How else can Peter get away with this for so long without his wife knowing? He would have created a scandal in the '50s had it been discovered that a hole in his crotch was cut out.

As more and more women, female doctors, lawyers fantasize of being strippers, men are jumping into the act. Claudia, who writes eloquently of a lover who was endowed with an enormous penis, says, "A favorite fantasy of his was to work as a stripper at a women's club. He just loved me worshipping his dick. He couldn't get enough. It's probably why the relationship didn't work. As talented as I am, I can't imitate a thousand cheering women."

Alex

I'm a forty-two-year-old with an MBA, and I have to say, it's a beautiful day for voyeurs. I can't see a tight pair of jeans from the front or the back or the graceful shape of a breast (small, medium, or large) without fantasizing myself fondling or licking their owner's pussy. But nothing's hotter than when I look at a beautiful woman, and she looks back the same way.

When I was five, my sister, who's two years older, asked me to pull down my shorts so that I could show my penis to her girlfriends. There must've been about seven or eight girls who seemed to make a circle around me. I happily obliged. They immediately laughed and screamed with disgust, like it was the most horrible thing they'd ever seen. I think in some part, this led to my belief that the penis is ugly to women.

Maybe to deal with this, I've had a fantasy since high school that women organize a "penis beauty pageant." I imagine the women admiring my penis and those of my fellow contestants, with some joking and catcalls but also with gasps of appreciation and acknowledgments of sexual desire based only on this exposure. (By the way, the women can only see our cocks, but we men are on the other side of the curtain.)

I imagine my cock ends up winning, and the women grab my cock, pulling me through the curtain so that they can see who I really am.

Tad

I'm a thirty-one-year-old professor, in good shape. In my classes, I see many beautiful young women every day, and from the way they dress, it's easy to imagine what they look like nude. I admit, I sometimes fantasize what they may have done sexually. How they make love. What they would look like spread-eagle with a cock thrusting into them. I have to dress for the job, but I've been told I have a nice butt, so I always take my jacket off at the beginning of class. When I'm writing on the board, I think about them checking out my buns. It makes the job more interesting.

One of my earliest memories is of me and my male cousins taking a bath. Suddenly, my sister and several female cousins opened the door, waited for us to scream, and ran away. I don't know why this has stayed with me, but I can't forget the excitement they got from seeing us naked.

We know that men love to watch. They get hard looking at sex in all its variations. I used to think the erect penis had everything to do with men's staring, like an arrow pointing the way. But as women's fashions have gotten skimpier by the season, men seem to have become more reluctant to give women their eyes. Perhaps it's just not politically correct, or is it also that men today compete with women in the workplace and often lose? Some, like Jamie, may be damned if they will be like men of the previous generations and give women their eyes. No more, "You look good enough to eat." Now it's, "You take my job and now you want me to look at you, give you the satisfaction of having won my attention, too? Fat chance!"

Jamie

Jamie is a fifty-three-year-old married man with an advanced degree in engineering. For the last twenty years, he has worked for a successful company run primarily by women. At first, he thought this would be fun, as he found some of the women very attractive. Now he says he would feel "disdain" to look at any of his bosses in a sexual way. He also says that he has had little success in sharing fantasies with any of the women he has ever slept with.

It is not original to say that mothers can inflict as much damage on their sons as their daughters by their own repressed ideas about sexuality. At a given moment when I was eleven, my mother walked into my room unannounced and caught me with cock in hand and delivered a stern warning in a very disapproving manner. Several years later, I began to realize the inhibiting effect of her reaction to my sexual development. I then developed an alternative fantasy of her walking in, telling me there was nothing wrong with it, watching me do it, and offering a few suggestions for greater pleasure, including placing my hand back on my cock, with hers on top to help me continue. I noticed she was licking her fingers as she left the room.

Over the years, I have masturbated almost daily, sometimes in a darkened movie theater as a teenager. I have used many images in my mind: lovers, events, sometimes videos and magazines. I have not had the fortune to be married to a sexually curious or adventurous woman. Though she is multi-orgasmic, getting her to put my cock in her mouth was a major event. I have been unable to interest her in masturbation— hers or mine. This is leading me to the point of wanting an affair or to find a woman who is willing to participate with me in any number of exciting things, but I'm quite concerned about the emotional attachment that might develop, not to mention the aftereffect if I was found out. On to one of my favorite fantasies:

Helena, my girlfriend, asks me to do her a favor, that it will take a couple of hours this evening. When I get to her apartment, she says that her seventeen-year-old niece needs our help, and we have to get over to her house right away. When we get there, we go right to a back bedroom. She asks me to sit down so that we can get ready. Naturally, I wonder what's going on when she says I need to put on a blindfold. When it's in place, and taped over the forehead and eyes so I can't see, she tells me why we're there. Her niece had been asking some questions about sex and boys a couple of weeks ago. Since she and her friends haven't seen a naked man or had any sexual experience, Helena says she volunteered to "demonstrate" me at their next slumber party so they can get a real close look. As Helena starts undressing me, I'm beginning to realize what kind of experience lies ahead. I ask her what she's going to do; she tells me not to worry, that I'll do just fine, and I'll be under her control the whole time. She suddenly handcuffs my hands behind me, saying it'll be better that way.

There is a lot of nervous laughter as she leads me into the room by the cock and tells them they're going to get a close look at a real set of balls. Helena invites questions, and one asks how it gets hard. Another wants to know how big it gets.

Helena turns me around and tells me to sit down and lay back—it feels like a low coffee table with a pillow at one end. I'm spread very wide. The stirring in my cock continues as Helena stretches it out and holds it up for them to see. She asks everyone to get real close so they don't miss anything.

The idea of six or seven females clustered around my cock is very exciting. Helena takes my cock into her mouth and a nip or two with her teeth really got me started as she lets it back out so the girls can see what's going on. I'm pretty stiff by now and feel Helena's hand take a familiar position on the shaft. She explains how to position the fingers for the best effect. She starts to stroke me up and down and shows how to hold it tighter or looser and how to speed up or slow down as it gets harder. Then, I feel her mouth again, and she sucks me deeper.

My cock is now fully erect and at attention. The girls comment about its size and want to know if it will hurt going into their pussies. Helena assures them there will be plenty of natural lubrication and suggests they check their pussies right now. There are a number of "oohhs" and "ahhs." Helena removes her blouse and skirt and encourages them to take off whatever they want. She asks if any of them want to try, and I *feel Helena place a girl's hand on my cock. She giggles how hard it is, and for the first time, I speak, telling her how good it feels.*

Another girl tries. Helena shows them how to keep me from cumming by squeezing my balls just hard enough to ease the tension. Then, she resumes stroking, and I ask her to please let me cum. She tells me I'm not ready yet and squeezes some more. Then, she shows the girls how to take each ball into their mouths and gently pull and suck on them. The girls squeal with delight.

I start to shout how badly I need to cum. Knowing I'm being exhibited and controlled is having an effect on my mind, not to mention my cock. I hear them gasp as it disappears into her mouth again and applaud as I try to push up into her mouth even deeper. I yell again for Helena to let me cum. The girls agree it's time, and Helena tells them the real good part is about to happen. I thrust in her mouth one last time and then pull out as I explode like the fourth of July.

Glenn

I'm a thirty-six-year-old single man, and though I have had to endure a lifetime of humiliation and pain resulting from having been sexually abused as a child by my mother, I am finally starting to come into my own as a sexual being and am enjoying it. It is a real turn-on to read women's private sexual fantasies.

A typical one of mine is being at the doctor's for a physical exam (my doctor is female, younger than me, and quite sexy) and getting an erection when she checks my genitals and/or prostate gland. I have never actually gotten an erection in a physical exam (I have tingles though) because I get so panicked and afraid of being re-abused that I go into a traumatic reaction and freeze up. It is the weirdest combination of excitement and pain. I am afraid it will happen in an exam. Some of these fantasies involve nurses who walk in or are party to the exam. For example, the doctor squats down to look at my genitals (this really did happen). But then I start to get a hard-on, especially as she checks my balls. On the actual occasion when she said she wanted to check the alignment of my balls, I thought she was making an excuse to ogle my cock, and that really turned me on inside. I keep getting intensely re-stimulated when I recall those words.

In the fantasy, I am getting pretty big and sticking out straight. She acts cool, but I can tell she's turned on, too, and when she tells me to turn around and spread my legs for a rectal exam, I get even hotter. She slips her gloved finger deep into my ass and strokes my prostate, at which time I casually mention that I am having some erection problems. She has me turn around and asks me to try to make myself erect, and as I turn, she sees I am already getting pretty big. She gets down close to my cock and reinserts her finger into my ass, tells me she needs to check the ejaculatory response, and has me pump my cock. (She offers me some lubricant.) But even though she is acting cool, I sneak a peek down and see that her other hand is under her smock, and she is secretly jacking herself off. I start to moan, she increases her rectal probing, and I start to ejaculate. And as she sees my sperm erupt from my cock, she moans and cums too.

Clayton

Clayton is a young black virgin. In his fantasies, he fucks only beautiful women with authority: a teacher in front of her class, an anchorwoman on camera.

Many people assume that black people are always fucking and, because of this, they are magicians in the bedroom. I don't discourage this belief. I mostly play along and let people assume what they will about my sex life.

In junior high, at a private school I attended, there was a teacher who was very well-built and angular. She wore revealing clothes that emphasized her great body. All the guys would joke that if you didn't fantasize about her, something was wrong with you. During class, she would wiggle her sweet little ass while putting notes on the board. When passing out papers, she would slightly bend over, letting students get a glimpse of her soft, large breasts. Erections occurred by the dozens. My friends and I usually had to wait several minutes before leaving the class. Her classes were among the favorites.

My fantasy begins with me being told to stay after class while the rest of the class and the whole junior high go out to lunch. I stay after as instructed. She tells me to wait in her room while she goes to the bathroom. While she's gone, I hide under her desk. She comes back in a few minutes to find the room empty. She shuts the door and walks to her desk to write me up for disobeying her. She sits down. I notice she isn't wearing any panties. I am captivated by how hairy she is and immediately begin to explore her with my tongue. Startled, she drops her pen and spreads her legs wider in response. Her cunt swells as it gets wetter. I push her chair back from the desk, revealing myself. She is shocked at first but gets more turned on, which leads her to her first orgasm.

I glance over, seeing several friends looking through the door window. They're clearly excited and give me a thumbs up, implying they'll keep a watch out.

I stand up and clear the desk. She throws me on the desk. I am so hard I'm in pain. She unbuttons my pants, exposing my virgin prick. I undo her blouse and unhook her bra. She mounts me. I can't believe how warm and moist she feels. I see my friends watching and smiling as she starts to thrust up and down. I fondle her breasts, causing her nipples to get hard.

Over and over, she tells me how underdeveloped my penis is and how lucky I am she is fucking me. I start to feel the buildup of cum getting ready to shoot out of my cock as she screams louder and louder. I look over through the tinted classroom windows to see my classmates returning from lunch. My friends at the door signal to hurry up. This excites me, making me cum inside her quicker. We quickly disengage and rush to put our clothes back on as my friends at the door hold off the other kids. The students finally walk in to find me seated at a desk and her at her desk. They sit down as she begins her discussion of human sexuality, which is chapter nineteen in our health books.

Daydreaming about the encounter we just had, I look over by her desk on the floor. On the far side, away from my classmates, I notice her black bra. I ask permission to be excused. While getting a hall pass, I pick up the bra and tuck it under my shirt. I smile as I leave the classroom, the rush to put the bra in my locker as a souvenir and proof my buddies and I will have of what I did.

Matthew

I'm a thirty-one-year-old lawyer with innumerable fantasies and endless variations, the likes of which would fill volumes. Some are raunchier than others; some are mild. For instance, I sometimes see an attractive woman, and I picture what her body would look like and how she would act if I got her hot enough to go with me into a public bathroom and let me suck her tits. (I have actually done this a couple of times.)

I would also like to see a really old man, sixty to seventy, get sucked off by and try to fuck a really young-looking teenage nymph. Likewise, I would like to see a barely post-adolescent mulatto boy fuck a wrinkly, skinny, yet slightly attractive old white bitch with long, gray, dry hair and bright red lipstick.

One thing I find truly exciting is a woman who loves to fuck; the age or shape of the woman is secondary to my excitement level if I perceive her as loving to get rammed by a hard dick. I love the thought of young, beautiful lesbians licking each other and sucking each other's breasts. One recurring theme I use a lot when I masturbate is turning on an older woman, forty-five to fifty years old or so. I like to think of such a woman, usually an older Asian, who is still sexually attractive, getting turned on by the thought of having sex with me, a younger man. I fantasize that she hasn't had sex in three or four years, since her husband died. And when she did have sex, it was mediocre because her husband had a small penis and he was not very passionate or sensitive to what turns a woman on. I get off seeing her give in to her lust. I love picturing this woman getting rammed by me from behind, hearing the slapping of my thighs against her ass.

One last thing I would like to tell you that I have done, which relates to my penis. As I have gotten in touch with my primal desires, I realize that at my most narcissistic level, I want all females, young and old, throughout the entire world to worship my beautiful cock. I want it to be adored and pampered and purred over. In keeping with this, I recently emailed some nude photos of myself to women I consider myself close to but with whom I have never had a physical relationship. I got a certain high knowing that they would unexpectedly open my email and be exposed to the sight of my mighty rod.

"Look at me, damn it! Look at me!" the exhibitionist's posture demands. There is in fact so much on display on the street, the bus, the subway, that sometimes potential voyeurs look away, refusing to loan their gaze. It's a buyer's market, and they're having a feast.

Anything that one can own or wear, from cars to Prada shoes, is wanted by men and women desperate to create a persona. People have always wanted to be envied, but the degree today is breaking thermometers. As Tad says, "I think in part that I am very envious of women's sexuality, the way men turn to look at them, gawk, whistle. I want women to do that to me." Envy is a mean emotion. Nothing good can be said of its nasty "grrrrrr." "Why you and not me?" But the exhibitionists, to feel alive, would rather be hated for what they own than to be invisible.

Women's nipples (forget the bra) abound, barely concealed by sheer fabric; the outline of the curled penis is meant to be seen and admired. Go ahead and stare, that is what they are there for, eye candy. Help yourself. Don't be embarrassed. The owner is being fed by your eyes.

By putting him- or herself in our line of vision, the exhibitionist has "caught us."

Sexual exhibitionism is, of course, the final shame barrier, meaning fantasies of being watched in the sexual act bring the biggest bang. Those of us who build to orgasm with the fantasy of exhibiting ourselves are playing with the primal Do's and Don'ts of childhood. You could say, for the man or woman who masturbates and/or enjoys sex while fantasizing an attendant audience, the voyeurs represent the forbidding parents. The power felt at defying parental/societal anti-sex rules, along with the thrill of doing "it" in spite of the onlookers, all this becomes kindling to the sexual pleasure.

I have a certain kinship with the exhibitionist. I choose to write about sex. I went for the subject, straight as an arrow, back in the '70s when the curtain was raised for what women could do, could show and be. While I've had success with my chosen subject, I took my share of abuse at the beginning, from my family, from certain friends, from the media. For better or worse, today, sex is front and center, selling everything from cars to paper towels.

FEMALE FANTASIES OF EXHIBITIONISM, OR,
"Open the Door—I'm Naked!"

Today, both men and women use everything to draw attention to themselves. Being seen, yes, even being envied for one's sexual beauty is not just allowed but sought after. The old parental admonitions, "Don't draw attention to yourself," and, "Don't stare," are seldom heard. "Yes, please look at me!" the fashions today cry out. With the sexual revolution came a release from inhibition. We are beautiful! Look at us!

I remember the opening night of the musical *Hair*, with which I was involved. The previous night, the discussion was whether the cast should drop their clothes and stand naked. The audience went crazy with delight when they did. Exhibitionism was in.

I built a life in defiance of my mother's disinterest in me. Very well, if you won't see me, I'll find others who will. And I did. Everybody in our little town loved me. But it came too late. It doesn't feed me. It doesn't get to the bedrock deep inside where I'm still invisible.

Today, without the loving eye that takes in the child, without the gaze holding them close that first year, then letting them go, he or she can feel invisible. We adults have had times in our lives when we too felt alone and invisible. Imagine how a child, who can't provide for him- or herself, feels when the frightening awareness of not being seen settles in.

Terry

I'm a thirty-three-year-old woman from an Australian town near Sydney. You asked for biographical details, and these I gladly supply. I have tried to identify why my sexual fantasies and whims are as they are by thinking back on past experiences in early life. My fantasies always seem to center on embarrassment, subjugation, humiliation, abuse, and, perhaps, exhibitionism. I also think that in some small way, they are masochistic, although I have never sought physical pain as such and, indeed, would probably shrink from it. But the threat of such pain, abuse, or misuse can easily turn me on.

I was brought up very strictly. My mother and father had separate rooms and separate beds, and I never saw or heard of any physical relationship they had together. My mother always impressed on me that my body was personal to myself and perhaps to my doctor—who should always be a lad. It should never, ever, be seen by anyone else. And from a very early age, I was taught that it was wicked to finger myself "there."

I never masturbated deliberately until I was in my late teens, although as early as twelve, I would sometimes close my legs very tightly together when thinking of something "wicked" and get a strange kind of relief.

My earliest sexual experience was when I made a visit to some relatives. We had some cousins who lived in the outback, and some of them came to visit us occasionally. The event which I believe started some of my fantasies occurred when bath night arrived. A large tub was brought into the kitchen and was filled with hot water for the family baths. As my uncle was the head of the family, it was the tradition—so it seemed—that he should bathe first, followed by the children and lastly by my aunt. I remember that I was partly terrified by the thought of what was going to happen and partly, I realize now, exhilarated by the prospect of "having no choice."

I had imagined that we would all be sent out of the kitchen whilst the bathing took place, but this was not so. My uncle arrived for his bath in his dressing gown, which he took off, and stepped into the tub. I had never, ever seen a man naked before and remember well his huge genitals, which protruded from the mass of black hair which he had between his legs.

It seemed as if my turn was next, as I was a guest, so I was asked to undress there and then and jump in the bath. I was quite terrified, but my younger cousin shouted hurry up—we don't have all day, and the water will get cold. So, I was about to get into the bath when my uncle said, "Let me see this little girl; she's beginning to grow up." I remember I tried to avoid him, but somehow my aunt said, "Come—don't be so shy, let your uncle see you now that you are undressed—like a proper big girl," and catching me by the arm, she pulled me so as to make me face him. "Yes, you are growing up nicely," he said and turning to my aunt said, "You see her breasts are starting to grow, and her nipples are harder now—and she has some hair between her legs." He touched me there on my hair and said, "Yes, fine, you'll be a really big girl soon." My uncle continued to dry himself, and as he did, and the towel parted, I noticed that his penis, which I had thought was huge, seemed to have become even bigger still.

The experience stayed with me but didn't traumatize me in any way—in fact, the reverse, for when I thought of it—as I often did—it seems to give me some sort of inner satisfaction, leading to a kind of sexual stimulation. Of course, I said nothing at all to my mother and father.

Three years passed before I revisited the outback. It was bath night again. This time, my aunt said I could undress in another room and wear a robe. I was a little disappointed at this. But when I came back and my uncle got out of the bath, I noticed that his penis had, this time, become almost erect. Being big in any case, he now seemed gigantic. For fear of being called a prude, I dared not cover myself with my hands as I got into the bath. My cousin was naked before I sat down, and I noticed how enormous he was between his legs and how he too had become quite erect. My aunt, seeing him, just said, "My, my, you seem to be disturbed by your cousin who has grown into a big girl."

These incidents stayed on my mind and fermented into one of the fantasies which makes me so sexually stimulated today—fantasies in which I am forced one way or another to be exposed to and be seen by people. A friend of mine at the university was turned on to some bits of bondage fantasies and told me he'd like to have me tied up and then "do whatever he wanted to me." I should've told him, "Go for it!" But I was too shy. It was with this same boy, however, that I first had oral sex after he asked me to suck him.

I'm now in a great marriage. I love everything about my husband except our sex life. It's very conventional. Sometimes, it leaves me unsatisfied. Sometimes, I need some fantasy to help me out.

I imagine that I live in a modern age but one in which women have neither rights nor redress. They are dependent on men and are required to obey their demands and instructions. It is in such an environment that I pretend that my husband decides to sell me and advertises me in the newspaper. Of course, I presume to be very upset that he doesn't want me, but he is quite severe and ignores my protestations.

He tells me he had an interested enquirer, who is coming to see me that evening.

A gentleman who is tall and big and perhaps fifty or more arrives. He is very elegant and well-dressed—like perhaps a diplomat. He is accompanied by his wife, who is younger than he but also elegantly dressed. She is about forty years old. There is also their son, whom they say is fifteen. He is wearing a tracksuit and trainers. My husband invites them into our big lounge, and immediately I am introduced. My husband is quite severe with me—treating me as chattel that he wishes to be rid of.

The lady then turns to my husband. She asks: "I take it there are no restrictions on the purposes for which we can use her? My husband has certain unusual physical needs that I find it hard to satisfy."

"I am sure she will suit you well," says my husband without showing concern.

"Before we firmly say yes, though, we would like to examine her more thoroughly," says the lady, "and perhaps that can be arranged."

I go to my room and strip. Then, totally nude but for high-heeled shoes, I return to the lounge. I feel terribly shy—even in front of my husband, for our life together has always been very discreet. I cover myself with my hands as I enter. I am terrified to be seen by these people and especially the young boy. "Come face this lady and gentleman," says my husband, "and let them see your figure. Put your hands behind your back so that they can see you properly." I have to obey, and as I stand there, I see the boy looking at me quizzically, and I see the bulge in the man's trousers as he surveys my body. The man then touches the top of my thighs and begins to push his finger between them.

"Stand with your legs parted," says my husband, "and let the gentleman examine you properly if he wishes." I do as I am told and *feel his fingers between my lips, and then as he slowly pushes one finger inside me, I squirm. The man stops and says something to his wife. She then asks my husband if I can lie on my back on a long coffee table we have in our lounge and open my legs and draw them up a little. My husband orders me to do so immediately. The lady then spreads open the lips of my vagina and calls her husband over to see my clitoris, which she touches lightly with her long red fingernail.*

"She has much too much hair here," she says. "Some of this will have to come off." I am then asked to stand again.

"Down on your elbows," my husband says, "and part your thighs slightly so that you can be seen properly." The man then fondles my big hanging breasts more roughly and moves onto my nipples, which he squeezes and pulls. I feel myself being opened at the back—the cheeks of my bottom being pulled wide apart and something cold touching my anus. I hear the lady open and then remove something from the inside of a vanity bag which she brought with her and then the cold end of something being pushed into my uterus. It is thick and long and fills me. It is then expanded somehow and fills me almost to the bursting point. I feel her touch my bottom again.

"She's fine for my husband in her vagina," I hear her say, "but her anus is too tight for him—he would split her, and I don't want the trouble of that. But I think she will do. I can have her anus checked and opened by some people I know." The young boy watches her intently as she takes that "thing" out of me, and I see his penis quite clearly outlined through his track suit and notice how erect is his apparently large organ. He puts his hand on the inside of the top of my thigh, but his mother pushes him away quietly, saying, "No, not now. You'll have lots of chance when we get her home."

It is plain as day to see the almost exact replication—with some additions—to the actual experience of taking a bath at her aunt's house, with everyone looking on.

Grace

The setting is a large bar, kind of country-western style. (I don't know why, as I am heavy metal all the way.) I am a hired "waitress." I waltz around the room, serving beers and liquor to the customers. Suddenly, I feel a hand snaking up my thigh. I notice that it isn't one of the "authorized" men, but I let him have his way for a few minutes. This gets me a little wet, but the next touch I feel is more aggressive; my tray is taken from me, and in the same swift motion, I am pushed down across one of the little tables and roundly fucked. I'm absolutely loving it, but they don't know that. The fact that I'm being paid to fuck these men is integral to the whole thing.

I understand the importance to the fantasy of being paid to fuck in public. It not only elevates the act to pure art, but at the same time, it gives roots to Grace's exhibitionism, making it as practical and worthwhile as tending bar or waiting on tables. After all, isn't she feeding the customers' eyes?

When feminism came along, women's pursuit of beauty was rejected. When women entered the workplace, the full asexual Dress for Success suit said, "Don't take me as a sex object. I'm here to compete." I don't recall any debate on the decision, but intuitively, we realized that we'd never forge an army if we were divided by envy of other women's beauty or stopping to powder our nose on the way to the march. We simply put on our jeans and went to war.

That era didn't last long. Once we'd won a piece of the economic pie, we "naturally" (if that word means anything) wanted to buy something lovely and go out and be seen. We kept our jeans, but we also wanted that deep-down pleasure in being taken. With men and women in a confined space, eros will find a way. Janet, a forty-two-year-old woman, unmarried but living with a man, writes: "My lover and I shared our fantasies with each other last night in a hotel room. As he was lapping up my cunt juices, I was fantasizing about a man I used to work with. I used to love the way he'd sneak glances at me. Though we never acknowledged it, I loved the power I had over him. I dressed to get more."

We can do what we want with people, put them into various configurations, workplace, home—but the need to see and be seen—both of which feed eros—demand gratification.

Risa

Risa is an attractive, fifty-year-old college professor.

I had a foreign student in one of my classes; he wore a short dress-like garment. He always sat in the front row, right where he made eye contact with me, no matter where I was lecturing. He began to move his legs open and closed very suggestively throughout the hour. I had no idea if he had underwear on or not. I finally asked him to take a seat in the back. He did but was clever enough to take a back seat which was, again, directly in my line of vision. I couldn't teach. I got through the semester, but my fantasies of him continue. It wasn't just that he was possibly exposing himself. It's that I was the focus of this sexual young man's exhibitionistic pleasure. I have to admit, the thought of it always heightens my orgasms.

On an intellectual level, I understand that it has very little to do with me. I was the one lecturing, the supposed focus, and he wanted/needed the eye on him. To some degree, we all want that. I remember when I was five, wearing a polka-dot bathing suit and a hula skirt for Halloween, and my teacher asking us to change into our clothes when we came in from the march outside into the classroom. I refused to take off my bathing suit and was conscious that I wanted the boys to see me.

We know that the intent of the display artist is to capture someone's eye and keep it, literally control it. Often, the voyeur is accused of staring, making the beautiful woman with the pushup bra in the transparent dress uncomfortable. The dilemma is that we want to get attention, to dominate the eye of another, but we also want to be the one in charge.

Stella

Stella, a twenty-year-old student at a prestigious university, is active in her sorority and other campus organizations.

Both my parents have remarried and returned to the church, and although they were pretty liberal while I was growing up, I find that now they would rather have me be "a good little girl." Perhaps this is one of the reasons sex is just a little more thrilling now, as I have always done what I was supposed to do.

I am currently seeing a twenty-six-year-old man with the body of a Greek god. It is hard for me to fantasize about a better body, so in my head and in real life, they are one and the same. My fantasy goes something like this: My lover and I plan to meet in a bar or perhaps he just knows that I will be there and wants to make sure that he is the man I'll be with for the evening. The bar is something out of an old movie, almost like a whorehouse bar with red satin walls and a big dark oak bar with a handsome bartender who serves me free drinks. I am at the middle bar stool alone, and the whole room is filled with a haze of smoke and men's laughter. Some men are playing cards, and others are just talking, but they all keep sneaking looks at me.

I am wearing a black formal evening dress with black lace stockings. I have no panties on, so I can feel the slipperiness of the satin beneath my ass when I cross and recross my legs. The smoky bar is warm, and I am thankful that my dress is short and strapless, since I can see the perspiration beginning to form across my chest.

When I look up from my drink, I see my lover come in the door. I smile, but he gives me a cool look. He walks up to the bar slowly, and as he gets closer, I can smell his clean, fresh-shaven scent. He sits down next to me and orders a strong drink, the whole time ignoring me as I am getting wetter and wetter just being near him. I turn my bar stool toward him, and my knees brush his pants. He can see all the way to my pink lips, and he can smell the heat of my cunt. Without looking at my face, he slides his hands slowly up my dress past the top of my stockings and begins to finger me. He turns slightly toward me and smirks, knowing how badly I want him.

The bartender comes down to offer me another drink. As I have trouble ordering another drink, he smiles, knowing what is happening. Meanwhile, I can see the bulge in my lover's pants, so I reach to unzip and free his throbbing desire. He clasps onto my wrist quickly, pulls his other hand out from my dripping cunt, and takes me to a dark hallway that leads to a pool room. The whole room of men can see us as he presses me up against the wall, both of my hands above my head held in one of his big strong hands, as he lifts up my dress, and pulls me, moaning, onto his hard shaft. He reaches under my ass to lift me from the floor, kissing me, and moves me to him until we cum together. Then, he pulls down my dress, kisses me gently, and we walk out of the dark saloon together, his juices flowing down the inside of my thigh.

Dixie

I'm a twenty-five-year-old black girl, middle class and single. I spent a wonderful summer with Joel, a boy about a year older than I. He's going to be married now, but I still sometimes fantasize about people, usually men, watching us have sex in unusual places.

At the Metropolitan Opera House, in the parking lot, are two bathrooms for men and women. I've often gone there and seen no one on duty. He doesn't know where we're going and looks surprised when I pull him into the men's bathroom. (I envision it has stalls like the women's room.)

There are several men in stalls, but no one sees us as we slip into one. Once inside a stall, we start hugging each other frantically. I tug at his shirt, popping off a few of the buttons in my hurry. He's wearing a T-shirt underneath and doesn't protest when I start tearing at it. It comes apart with a satisfying ripping sound. I can sense this gets the attention of the men in the stalls. I feel like an animal; I'm different from how he's always seen me. He's inspired by my hunger, carried away by lust. Abandoning restraint, he pulls down the top of my dress; I'm wearing one of those black lace skimpy bras underneath. He flicks his tongue all along the edge of the bra, even sucking my nipples through the lace.

The men in the stalls begin looking over the top to see what's going on as Joel pulls my bra down with his teeth, leaving it in tangles, almost pinning my arms. We don't have much time, as more and more men come in. They are now looking from over and under the stall. Joel's erection presses into me with one sudden thrust, causing me to cry out. I'm not quite wet enough for him yet, so he has to shove harder than usual to move into me. But I don't mind—it's what I want. Standing up, there's barely room to move. I see men all around lustfully staring as Joel fucks me. The constrained space means we're banging against the walls, arching our bodies together, slippery with sweat. My legs are wrapped tight around his waist; he couldn't throw me off even if he wanted to. I want to have his cock deep inside me. He silences me with a kiss, but his thrusts become even fiercer, if possible, as the men are now cheering him on saying, "Fuck her! Screw that hot bitch!"

I reach down and rub his cock when it partly comes out of my cunt. I bring up my fingers, dripping with my own juice, and smear my nipples with it. I'm gasping, nearly sobbing with pleasure. Through the men's voices cheering him on, I hear him groaning out my name: now he's just groaning. I twist against him and feel orgasms shuddering through me. Finally, he cums, his stiffened body grinding me into the stall door as the huge crowd of men cheers. We wipe each other's bodies with the toilet paper and slip quietly out of the bathroom before the guards get there to find out what all the commotion is about.

MALE FANTASIES OF VOYEURISM
"Peekaboo," or, "Pass the Remote"

I remember the thrill when I was a young child of "spying" on people. There was a game of following strangers on the street, ducking in and out of doorways, keeping them in our gaze as if it were an exercise of power. We learn not to be caught staring at someone, to not want to be seen. "It's impolite," Mother says. But it's hard not to look. We are wired to gaze at beauty. We are hungry for it: "Let me take you in. Let me feast my eyes!" Even if we're envious, we can't resist a peek.

We criticize, try to find some defect. When you are rich in beauty, you experience all the pros and cons of your wealth. When love, real love, is offered, many beautiful people don't believe it any more than the very rich believe they are loved for themselves.

Eddie

I have been married now for six years. We have no children yet. I want one or two, but my wife has changed her mind and now wants none. We may have to divorce over this irreconcilable difference. We have a repertoire of four positions. I believe my early childhood experiences helped mold the strong voyeur streak in me. When I lived in my parents' house, until I was twenty-five, I could see across to another apartment, where this incredibly hot neighbor was having frequent sex in a lesbian relationship.

In one of my fantasies, I am never present. It is like a porno flick in the making, and I am a roving cameraman who picks up the sights, sounds, smells, and sensations of the scent. This scenario has been developing and evolving over the years.

A large mansion resort, à la Playboy Mansion, is built surrounded by a large expansion of well-tended and groomed fields and meadows with skinny-dipping ponds, a small cave, a man-made waterfall, etc.

Farther out is an evergreen forest to keep out trespassers. Access to the resort is by a paved road that is barred with a gate and a large guardhouse/cottage. Guests arrive and check in with the two beautiful female guards at the guardhouse cottage. The guests undergo a medical checkup to screen for STDs (sexually transmitted diseases). First-time guests are briefed on the house rules. They are as follows:

All guests can wear at most is one layer of clothing. Partial or total nudity is at the guest's discretion. The gorgeous, mostly female house staff also wears only one layer of clothing or uniform and cannot refuse any sexual request from a guest except for anal sex. The female staff also wears either a bracelet or a necklace. The color code immediately indicates if the woman is agreeable to anal sex or not. This option is overruled under provisions described in another house rule.

Male staff do not engage in homosexual acts under any circumstances.

Sexual acts can be done anywhere, anytime, alone, or in groups.

A guest can refuse a sexual request from another guest.

If a guest witnesses one person masturbating or witnesses a couple fucking, the proper etiquette for joining in is to approach the people involved and begin to masturbate. If the person masturbating or the couple fucking wishes to be left alone, they will politely ignore the newly masturbating guest. Otherwise, the joinee will be caressed into joining the sex act already in progress.

If three or more people are engaged in sex, it is open season to join in. For example, if a male guest sees a trio engaged in sex and develops an erection and a female in the group has her ass in the air, it is up to the male's discretion if he fucks her cunt, if he fucks her ass, fingers her clit, feels her tits, etc.

There are no restrictions on lesbian sex. In fact, it is encouraged.

The resort has a full-fledged library, several game rooms, with gambling games. Other game rooms have pinball machines and the very popular pool tables, and there is a bowling alley. The resort has a set of reward and punishment fortune cookie jars. (I always thought that a fortune cookie looked like a shaved cunt.) The guest can engage in any of the games with the added stakes that either the winners can pick up a reward fortune cookie or the losers get to dip into the punishment cunt jar.

Some of the women's punishments are: she must masturbate three guests, with at least one being a woman. She will be provided a chamber pot and must pee in public while nude.

Some of the women's rewards are: the nearest person to you will eat your cunt to your satisfaction or you can have sex with the guest of your choice. Similar prizes are in the men's jar.

I can reuse this fantasy framework over and over by simply building a fantasy based on various guests' escapades during their stay at the resort. This is an X-rated "Fantasy Island" without Ricardo Montalban or The Hobbit.

It is not just beauty we look for. Some things never change. Men are still wildly charged by fantasies of watching women losing all control sexually. As long as men are raised by women, this will be true. The dream of women *losing* control is thrilling. It takes her off the pedestal, making her supremely fuckable.

Men stagger out from under women's maternal rule, only to find themselves brought to their knees by the beauty of young girls who have all the power in the world to reject the hungry boy. Once again, the beauty of the breast enters his life, this time around feeding his eyes, tempting his hands, a mouth-watering kind of hunger different from the first time around.

In a few more years comes the workplace, where the breast's pre-eminence, far from fading, will be reinforced by the woman who uses her breasts, buttocks, whatever it takes to beat the guy out of the job. She will deny she is using her body to get ahead, but her heart won't be in it. "Business is cutthroat. You use what you've got to get the job," says my friend Sharlene.

Carl, a PhD and scientist, imagines a woman on a powerful aphrodisiac. His excitement comes from watching her lose all control during wild orgasm. Much as he may love women, no boy really ever gets over the feeling of total control a woman once had over him. How often he failed her expectations of him. Now he is watching a woman in the throes of orgasm, self-control gone with the wind. Oh, God, how marvelous to see her out of her mind in an orgasmic high!

NARCISSISTIC VOYEURISM

Instead of just looking, we find men today in front of the mirror as never before in modern times.

Carl

Besides watching a woman in an out-of-control orgasm, I love watching myself cum. My early masturbation was very experimental. I wanted to know how everything worked. I tried my best to pee while cumming (never could), shit while cumming (did but not easily), sneeze in the middle of orgasm (the feelings just stopped, but the ejaculation continued), hold my hand over my opening so the cum wouldn't come out (the pressure was too high; it just sprayed out like when you try to hold your thumb over the end of a hose. When I held it really hard, it didn't come out, but the tube got very sore for a while), get right to the brink of orgasm and see what sorts of stimulation will set me off. Once I got right to the brink, then put on tight pants and walked around in front of a mirror until the friction triggered orgasm. I still jerk off in front of the mirror.

When we imagine in fantasy an audience applauding, as in Alex's "biggest, most beautiful penis" contest, this adds genuine narcissism to the scene, a wish to be admired for one's sexual prowess, for one's body, the ability to be free, uninhibited. It is indeed raising oneself to the level of a performer. The narcissistic element, added to the erotic, doubles the sexual pleasure. In the first case, it is the power element: "*You*, my parent or society—watch *me*! I defy you!" And in the second case, it's the narcissistic element that increases sexual pleasure.

In the psychoanalytic world, the "audience" of lookers can represent the daydreamer him- or herself. Imagine this kind of double effect: the fantasizer is both a "peeper" as well as a performer.

The gorgeous male steps in front of the female. From his sheer trousers, one can see the detailed configuration of his penis. What a feast for the eyes! But who is looking? The hot blonde with the breast implants? The dreamy boy toy with the tanned, waxed chest? As the power of beauty sits more equally in both camps and the unrelenting competition to be seen and admired shrinks the audience, do mirror sales increase?

Lora

Lora, a virgin, feeds her eyes with the image of herself masturbating in front of all the mirrors in her house. Leave no glass unfilled!

I lived with my parents until I was twenty-five, and starting from when I was seventeen, if my parents were out of town or just not home, and I would get real horny, I would masturbate in front of all the mirrors in the house. (Our house had lots of mirrors.) It turned me on just watching myself masturbate. I'd pretend that my image was really into me watching, really getting turned on by it. Sometimes, I'd pretend that my image was into watching me, but that was harder to do.

At the age of thirty-one, I'm still a virgin, and the following is my newest fantasy: Desperate to lose my virginity, I decide to run a personal ad online:

> *THIRTY-ONE YEAR OLD ARIES FE-*
> *MALE WHO WISHES TO LOSE HER*
> *VIRGINITY AND SATISFY BUILT-UP*
> *ENERGIES LOOKS FOR PARTIES TO*
> *ASSIST HER IN ACHIEVING THIS GOAL.*
> *IF INTERESTED, PLEASE BE AT (my*
> *address) ON 4-4 (my birthday, too. Oh, what a*
> *present!) THE DOOR WILL BE OPEN, JUST*
> *WALK IN AND SHE WILL BE READY!*

The line of thousands of men waiting to fuck me goes all the way to the state line, and they all get satisfied by me.

I relate to Lora's determination, honoring and applauding her efforts to reflect her own sexuality.

FEMALE FANTASIES OF VOYEURISM, OR,
"Why's a Nice Girl Like You Hiding in a Place Like That?"

It's exciting to see women getting into voyeurism! When I think of the amount of sexual "needs" women swallowed so as to fit the stereotype of patriarchy prior to the '70s, I'm amazed how we lived with it. Believing that women weren't sexually aroused by visual stimuli was passed from mother to daughter. It's amazing it worked, considering the amount of industry today that feeds women's eyes, turns us on, makes us hot and eager to masturbate or find a partner.

What a lopsided world we used to have in which half the human race was supposed to feel nothing when they looked at nudity or blue movies or the naked person bedside them in bed.

When I was twelve, I remember some of the older women in Charleston complaining to authorities on a hot summer day that sailors were working on decks of ships with no shirts on. The culpable sailors were promptly dealt with. I told everyone how unfair I thought it was that the sailors should have to work in such extreme heat with their shirts on. But the real anger came from not being allowed to see their gorgeous, stripped torsos. It was a pleasure I felt entitled to. What was the great fear of these ridiculous women?! Could this lack of propriety really taint their despicably pure eyes?! I realize now that the answer is an astounding, "Yes!"

How difficult it must have been for women back then to suppress lustful thoughts, especially with these bare-chested Adonises strutting practically in front of their faces. How it must have threatened their tightly held nonsexual conceptions of themselves.

When I look back, I realize how much these women gave up to support a false image, a lie. All to be accepted, to assure mother's love. It's all well and good being the exhibitionist, getting oneself seen, taken in, visually adored, feeling the warmth of eyes: "Let me look at you. Let me take you in. Dear God, you're a sight for sore eyes, and mine adore you!" But voyeurism is an equally charged flip side of this coin. How lovely it is nowadays to take in and admire the male body, as delicious eye candy as a woman's body.

As for the flashing man, an unsettling moment, that's a different matter. It isn't just the sight of a flasher's penis that upsets us but that he has captured our eye and, for a moment, held it. He has involved us in this nasty act. Forced us to mentally participate. A woman feels insulted, afraid, angry. Is the anger because the flasher's penis isn't big enough, beautiful enough? No, he's forced us out of our state of innocence, the state where we have mother's approval, leaving the unintended voyeur with a little nightmare of a scene she's unlikely to forget. As for the flasher, getting a frightened, angry reaction from a woman says "I am powerful!"

The flasher is a man who feels inadequate, doesn't measure up in his own eyes. By grabbing a woman's attention and causing an emotional avalanche, he feels powerful. It is a form of visual rape. Once, when I was a little girl, a man flashed his penis at me. I was terrified.

Before going online, Joyce felt she was one of the only women who enjoyed looking at the naked male body. Joyce had the frightening experience of having men expose themselves to her. However, her fantasies of looking at a handsome guy "strip and masturbate for me, is very hot—the hotter he gets, the more excited I get because the more I feel in control."

Roz

One of the changes I heartily embrace is women's voyeuristic fantasies of watching their men masturbate. Roz, a young housewife and mother, scoffs at the idea that women are the exhibitionists.

My husband is the focal point of most of my fantasies. I love to think about him masturbating. I once walked into the bathroom while he was in the shower. The shower door is frosted glass, and I could tell he was beating off. He was embarrassed when he realized I was there, but I was incredibly turned on by it. Once I told him that, he relaxed. And now the bathroom door is always wide open when he showers.

In one of my fantasies, I imagine it's late at night, and I wake up to realize my husband isn't in bed with me. I hear noises in the living room and quietly creep out to see what's going on. He's lying on the couch, naked, watching a dirty movie. He doesn't notice me standing there, and I watch as he softly strokes his penis, almost teasingly, until he can't stand it anymore. I'd also like it if he had a wet dream while I was lying next to him in bed awake.

Unlike the women who loathe feeling unnecessary, a terrifying emotional state if you're dependent, Roz doesn't mind knowing that other women turn on her husband. She loves that he is so sexual that he masturbates. It implies that women are getting more sexually secure, a profound coming of age for women. This is what men used to say about watching women masturbate—loud and clear, it said that they love sex.

When men had all the power—money—and women took care of home and family, a successful man "wore" his lovely wife as a token of his professional standing. His wife spent his money to beautify herself and/or their children and home. There was little sexual content in his display, and whatever subliminal pleasure this picture might convey, its roots were conventional.

Women, and men, may have gone in droves to see an almost-naked Douglas Fairbanks or Johnny Weissmuller, but sexual gratification from seeing these bare-chested movie stars wasn't taken seriously. There weren't shades-of-gray distinctions. It was absolute that we women weren't interested in watching erotica. Is it a coincidence that once we could pay the rent, women became watchers? Which, of course, we'd always been.

Charlotte

I'm a twenty-four-year-old receptionist and lead a relatively normal life. But I'm a very creative person with an active imagination. I fantasize about living in the Golden Age of Greece. My king and I are constantly in comfort, being caressed by both male and female slaves. The slaves often fight over who bathes him, being he is so incredible in every way. His eyes are closed as the women run their soapy hands over his long, lean body. My desire for him rises to a high degree of heat. The longer I watch him, the more my desire grows. I must have that beautiful penis inside me!

Most of my fantasies also involve one of the men being a father figure to a younger one. Here is one of them: A young man is watching TV on the couch. Enter an older man, possibly a friend of the family. He has come to the house because a snowstorm has prevented him from making it back to his house. They are alone in the house for the remainder of the storm.

As the day goes on, feeling a little frisky, the younger man starts to wrestle with the older man. They both enjoy pouncing on each other when all of a sudden, the younger man becomes too violent. The older man gets angry and yells for the other to stop. He puts him on the floor and reprimands him. The young man mimics the other and receives a slap in the face. He starts to cry and begs to be let go. Once free, he pushes the older man to the floor and runs to his bedroom. The older man runs after him and demands that he apologize. When he refuses, the older man grabs him and pulls off his clothes. He tells him that he is going to get the strap for talking back. The older man takes off his belt while pushing the younger man facedown on the bed. He starts to whip his naked bottom with the strap. The young man cries out in pain and begs for the other to stop. The older man tells him he needs to learn some respect.

Later that evening, the older man comes into the young man's room again. The young man is still crying from being spanked so hard. The older man comforts him by sitting next to him and stroking his head. This eventually turns into something more sexual. They both start to hug and kiss each other. The younger man takes the other's penis in his mouth and sucks it until he is good and hard. The older man then positions him bent over the edge of the bed. He then enters him after pouring body oil on his penis and massaging some over the younger man's bottom and anus. He starts to pump faster and faster. This goes on for quite some time. They both start to yell and scream in complete joy. They both ejaculate at the same time and fall to the bed, completely exhausted. Meanwhile, the storm continues outside the window. This is one of my favorite fantasies.

We are in high flux sexually. Where men and women are concerned, there are no longer any absolutes. Economically, professionally, we are inkblots, spreading, merging. Thirty-five years ago, it was rare to come across women fantasizing about two men having sex. Julia, who is thirty, like many women now, loves to masturbate to gay porn sites. Even offline, she fantasies watching "two guys doing it." Sometimes, she enters the fantasy as a guy or—why not?—"a sleazy goddess."

We understand that many men are aroused at the sight of women lying in one another's arms. It's nice to see that women are now finally secure enough to partake in the fun. Unfortunately, I'm from the old school. When I try watching two men having sex, what I feel is "left out." Much as I love my gay male friends, I wouldn't want to see them having sex. It is not because I'm repulsed by them—far from it. It is because I know that I will be on the outside looking in.

It's good to see young women today, like Brooke, Julia, Alicia, have moved past this feeling, forging ahead.

Alicia

Alicia, a law student in love with a gay man, fantasizes watching the object of her desire fuck another man.

I realize it's pathetic, but if I can't have him in reality, I'll join him and my rival in a fantasy threesome. I met my husband in college, and mostly because of parental pressure, we got married. The marriage unraveled quickly, and I stopped fantasizing about him. Then, I met

Gary, another law student. We hit it off immediately, and I was very attracted to him, even though I was married and there didn't seem to be much hope. Eventually, I decided to separate from my husband, and fantasies of Gary looked like they were going to come true. He was very attentive to me. This pattern continued for a full year, until a month ago, when he finally told me that the problem was he's gay.

From a fantasy point of view, all this puts me in a quandary. I want to stop fantasizing about him because it only makes it worse. I know him so well that I can even imagine how his face looks when he cums. It excites me to imagine a man doing this to him because I know that's what he likes. I want him to gaze at me and be excited that he could do that to me.

I spy on Gary as he sleeps on his back on a deserted beach in the sun. His body is oiled, and he is wearing black shorts and sunglasses. Our mutual friend, Mort, whom I know Gary would not be averse to fucking and who may be gay or bi (for all I know), comes along and catches me watching Gary. I tell Mort I was just waiting for Gary to wake up so that I'd have someone to swim with. Mort says he'll swim with me, and as we enter the water, we start pushing each other around and laughing. Eventually, the playing becomes sexual, and we fling our wet bathing suits onto the shore next to Gary, who wakes up and sees us but doesn't move. Mort touches me sensuously, running his hands over my ass and breasts. The whole time, I'm keeping an eye on Gary, watching him, waiting to see if I get a reaction. I take Mort's hard, wet penis in my hands, and he groans. We continue exploring each other slowly, still in the water.

Eventually, we move to drier land. I keep looking over to see if Gary has noticed us. His sunglasses hide his gaze, and he isn't moving, but a large bulge fills his shorts. Mort and I are on a towel some distance from Gary, and Mort goes down on my pussy, kissing and nibbling my clit, *making me moan. Finally, Gary can't stand it and comes over to where we are, naked and with his prick in his hand, rubbing slowly. We invite him to lie down with us, and he gives us each a kiss (this is not a problem for Mort in my fantasy!). We all get tangled up together, me and these two men I care about. The fun doesn't end until I have given them each a blow job and then Gary fucks me while Mort fucks him in the ass.*

I have seen them suck each other's pricks and swallow the other's load while I contentedly masturbate and attend to any parts of their bodies which need special attention.

I sometimes wonder if the world will hold together long enough to see how this relatively new emergence of women's sexuality pans out. An old friend just called to tell me he is working on an exhibition that will open in Russia. "It's about women pilots in World War II," he said and added, "Some of the women were so good that men tampered with the equipment on their planes, causing them to crash, killing several of the women."

How could men's fear of women be so profound that even during war, when it was so desperately needed, they would still resent the excellence of women's work in a man's job? Again, there is no answer but that the roots go back to the beginning of men's lives when they were totally controlled by a woman, their unconscious knowledge of the power women can have.

In fantasy, young women today like to play with domination, where they get hot holding the reins tightly and making the plot gallop just where they want it to go. Sometimes with them on top, then, quick as the snap of a whip, they are enslaved.

Vanessa, a twenty-six-year-old woman, tells me of the joy at being a "late bloomer. When I finally got my looks, how I loved the power I had over men. I really held back when I was younger, but now in my fantasies and in reality, I make men give me the sex I desire. I make them strip. I make them show themselves to me. In fantasyland, they are all mine—and their submission to me is on my terms."

Women becoming sexually secure has everything to do with being able to take care of oneself and another person too. If a woman isn't earning money on her own, she may fear the worst; meaning, she would die if he acted on his fantasy and actually left her for his fantasy woman. But women today also know that if the worst happens, it's possible for them to get a job, pay the rent, put food on the table. It's the *knowing* that matters, knowledge our grandmothers didn't have. There were so few women with economic independence in the past.

Can you ever totally separate money from sex? Perhaps it's easier done than with "love." At some level, money plays into domination/submission. It can get you laid and can emotionally empower you to invent the seduction. Anastasia's fantasy of being the headmistress gives her the power to control, to be the ruler of her sexual world.

Anastasia

I'm a twenty-three-year-old virgin who just graduated from a California university, and this has become my favorite fantasy:

I'm a headmistress at an exclusive girls' school. I'm both loved and feared; I maintain a friendly and close relationship with my students, but everybody knows I won't tolerate any infraction of the rules. I love my job because I get to look at beautiful, blossoming young women in the uniforms I have specifically selected for them: very tight sweaters emblazoned with the school crest, short plaid kilts that barely cover their crotches, knee socks, and saddle shoes.

I am especially turned on by one student named Esther (based on my real coworker), who is a voluptuous blonde with innocent brown eyes and full lips that always have a smile for me. I am bound and determined to initiate her into the joys of lesbian sex, but I don't know how. Besides, I'm worried about my job—she is, after all, only seventeen, and I could get into a lot of trouble. So, I content myself with finger-fucking at night and dreaming about her.

Then, one day, my assistant comes rushing into my office. She is a gorgeous black woman that I fantasize about on rare occasions when I'm able to put Esther out of my mind. She tells me, in a shocked voice, that Esther has been caught masturbating in the showers. I thunder, "Bring her to me!" and she runs off to get her.

When she returns, I ask her to leave, and Esther sits down. I say in my gentlest voice, "Now, Esther, I heard you were doing impure things in the bathroom." She is so embarrassed that she has tears in her eyes. I tell her to follow me to my bedroom so no one will ever overhear our private conversation, and she meekly follows.

I sit down on my bed and tell her to show me what she was doing. She is horrified and protests. I say, "Now, Esther, I can call your parents or we can resolve this here." Quickly, she sits down on the floor and spreads her legs, revealing her tiny, pristine white panties. A small spot of moisture is seeping through the crotch. She pulls the panties off, and I get my first, long-awaited look at her perfect little cunt. It is so tight that I can barely even see the opening, and her clitoris is the size and color of a tiny rosebud. She begins to rub herself, tentatively at first, blushing the entire time. Soon, she is so excited that she forgets where she is and throws her head back in abandon. Her cunt is getting wetter and wetter and finally she explodes in an incredible orgasm.

When she is finished, I say, "Esther, it's time for your punishment. Climb over my knee." She does, and I pull up her kilt to show her round buttocks. I begin to spank her, just hard enough to sting a little, and they get pinker and pinker. I am cumming just touching her, and as I continue, her legs are spreading and her already-wet pussy is getting wetter and opening up. Finally, she can't stand it, and she pulls up her sweater so she can fondle her tits as I spank her. When I'm done, my knee is wet from her cum and from my own juices. I finally say to hell with it and pull her dripping snatch onto my face. She is so sweet it is like her cunt is producing honey. I widen her tight little hole with my probing tongue and then she cums, humping my face with abandon.

I stand up, wipe my mouth on my sweater sleeve, and walk over to the phone. I call my assistant, Rhonda, and ask her to bring me "the rod." Esther is sitting on my bed with her legs splayed out, idly rubbing herself. "Are you going to spank me again?" she asks shyly.

"No, this is even better," I say, going over to kiss her. Rhonda lets herself in, and she's carrying a strap-on dildo that's at least eight inches long. Esther's eyes widen at the sight of it, and she licks her lips with nervous anticipation as Rhonda helps me strap it on.

"Esther, you better get down here and suck it, and you better get it really nice and slick because it's going inside of you." She falls to her knees in front of me and takes the whole cock into her mouth. I begin to think she's not as innocent as I originally thought. She looks up at me as she sucks it, and the sight of the huge rubber cock going in and out of her pink lips is enough to make me dizzy with desire.

Finally, the dildo is slick enough, and she gets down on her hands and knees on my bed. She looks over her shoulder at me, tossing her hair back and spreading her legs wider. "Come on, mistress. Give it to me—give it to me good!" she cries. I turn on the vibrating mechanism (which gives me a buzz, too) and jam the dildo into her cunt. She cries out and bites my pillow. I grab her hips and pump, thrusting into her, and she is calling my name, and I'm calling hers, and we cum over and over again. Meanwhile, Rhonda has started fucking herself with a candle, and that just sets me off on another wave of orgasms.

When we're finally too exhausted to keep cumming, we collapse in a heap on my bed. I send Rhonda on her way (with a promise to let her join us next time), and Esther unstraps the dildo and gently licks away my juices, not in an attempt to further stimulate me (there's only so much I can take!) but to clean me up. We fall asleep in each other's arms, and the next morning, we 69 each other, take a hot bubble bath together, fuck again, and I send her off to her afternoon classes with a very special hall pass. I tell her to use the pass any time she needs to "talk."

Between the exhibitionist and the voyeur, there is a kind of dance of domination, a power play, again, in fantasy and fact, the thrilling sensation of "holding, controlling" someone's gaze or "capturing them in your gaze to the point where they feel helpless and caught."

Being raised by a mother who didn't see me ignited both my exhibitionistic and voyeuristic needs. To a large degree, I have her to thank for my life. My need to be seen has been a driving force. It encouraged me to take chances, to go out into the world, to study sexuality in a way that would not have been possible had she been a doting mother and I her obedient daughter.

By defying my mother, refusing to be like her, I was able to study, discover who she and I really were behind our façades. What I ended up finding were striking similarities that I hadn't predicted. At a sexual level, though my efforts may have been more overt, my mother and I both needed, and equally worked, to be seen. And though I had difficulty admitting it, she and I shared a deep fondness for men, their company, their looks, and, yes, their devotion to us.

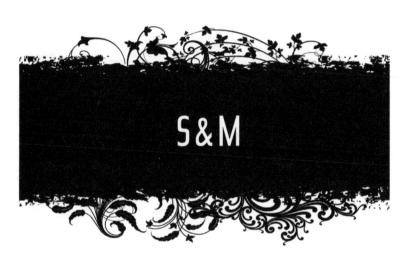

S&M

S & M

Fantasies of being forced into sex, made to spread our legs and take it—whatever "it" is that we desire—frees some women, and yes, men too, to relax their iron constraints and let go. Many of us don't have the slightest idea just why we can't give ourselves over to orgasm, but then, who can recall what got between us and the pleasure principle? Because Mother was the one we depended on for life itself and because we had to believe she loved us with all her heart, given that she was our whole world when we were most dependent, we don't punish Mother. Instead, we punish ourselves for wanting sex. In fantasies of sadomasochism, we are "bad, bad, bad" as we soar up into orgasm.

Only in erotic images of being held down and punished can some men and women allow themselves the forbidden sex they crave. The roots are too deep, the anti-sex tyrant of the nursery too rooted to be overwhelmed by the permission-giving, societal kiss of marriage. Oh, no, the celebration of marriage is in direct opposition. We prefer our sex in the dark, our copulation dirty, the forbidden stranger, and if it helps to oil the way to orgasm, throw in some arm-twisting, the lash of the whip, and, if you must, go ahead and "tie me up, lay me down!"

To find the forbidden fruit in the marital bed, we conjure up a daring, death-defying act of stolen sex. The brute inflicts the punishment that brings on that blessed first rush of orgasm. Perhaps, though in real life brutes still tend to be the males, it is no longer in any way a prerequisite. Included in this chapter are many submissive men, to show our changing tide, though a guy may want to be careful when invited up to the apartment of a woman after only an online chat.

MASOCHISTIC FANTASIES OF VIOLENT RAPE, OR,
"Where's a Dark, Dangerous Alley When You Need One?"

For many women and men, the rape fantasy is the sole means that works. In the masochistically experienced sexual act behind closed eyelids, we not only permit ourselves sexual satisfaction but at the same time pay for the guilt we experience through pain. Ergo, the fantasy serves a double purpose, which is why some derive orgasmic pleasure only with fantasies where they can hear their bones cracking. Enjoying the punishment with the sex is the down payment for orgasm. What most of us would experience as intolerable suffering, the aficionado of S&M finds within the pleasure range.

To fly to the heights of orgasm, why do some of us require fantasies of sadism, others masochism, others a mix of both, while others, even after growing up in this violent world, derive no thrill from thoughts of inflicting or receiving pain? The answer is unknown. Neither Polly nor Fauzia, the next two testimonials, were ever hit by their parents, yet their masochistic fantasies are their most exciting, most satisfying. Even if we haven't experienced parental abuse, it's possible for our minds to fill the gaps.

It wasn't long ago that a spanking was the accepted form of discipline. Corporal punishment may be greatly reduced today, but the threat is always present. Children see their parents angered over something they've done. What absolute guarantee is there that the rage won't be unleashed, physically turned against the child? No matter how loving, how caring, our parents are all-powerful. If pushed too far, we know we will inevitably suffer some form of their disappointment and anger.

We used to love to roughhouse, to be thrown in the air, swung around in ecstasy. Who cared about possibly getting hurt? The thrill was more than worth it. And at times, while roughhousing with other children, smaller and bigger, someone ended up injured, crying. Years later, how did those impressions affect us? When we brought a weaker opponent to tears, perhaps we felt remorse, feared getting into trouble, but at some level, we also feel the rush, the excitement, the thrill of power.

We could rule by force this person who, in some ways, may even be our superior. In our turn, when forced into submission by a larger hand, we felt our tears control them. It may have started out as a game, but they hurt us. They would have to live with what they had done. Their guilt would keep them in our power. Wrapped in these innocent childhood memories are seeds of our sadomasochistic fantasies waiting for whatever nutrients are needed to make them grow.

Polly

A young fledgling actress in the Midwest, Polly says she wasn't able to achieve orgasm until she was twenty.

My best friend called me and told me she had finally had an orgasm. We were both crazy for a while, doing it several times a day for weeks and just because we could. I've had nine lovers, mostly within a sort of relationship. And I've also made love with five women. I love women's bodies, but for me, guys are where it's at. I'd love to have two men on me, and I've been in a three-women/one-man bondage thing—great! I was never hit by my parents. I have two older brothers who would sometimes play rough with me, but I was never sexually abused. So, I don't know why fantasies like this are the ones that really get me going. I know I wouldn't want it to happen in real life.

I'm at a party, in a fancy house, looking very sexy. It's a good hair day. I go to the bathroom, and while I'm sitting on the stool, touching myself, getting really hot, a man walks into the stall.

He has a musky, sweet smell, green eyes, full, soft smiling lips. He tells me he overheard me outside talking with a friend sizing up what we think each guy's cock is like. I tell him it's not polite to eavesdrop. He tells me then he has to pee. I say go ahead. He laughs, like I'm crazy. He unzips his pants, allowing his beautiful tan penis to slip out, and releases a stream of urine between my legs while I'm still sitting on the commode. A little of it splashes on my thighs. He finishes and drops his pants the rest of the way. He plunges his fingers inside me, and I cry out. Then, he leads me upstairs in search of a little privacy.

As we walk into the room, he locks the door, and I see two other men inside. My heart beats with fear as I realize I'm trapped. They pull me to the bed, violently tear off my clothes, and tie my arms with neckties. I'm too scared to cry and still really aroused. They all strip and have huge beautiful cocks, all of them wanting me. The guy who brought me in there lies naked over me. He lowers his mouth to my vulva and quickly plunges his tongue inside of me. His tongue goes lower, stroking my behind and my rectum. The other two men straddle me. They're rock hard. One of them is stroking his cock in my face. He begins slapping my face hard with it. He begins to buck hard, moaning loud and licking his lips until I can see the cum shooting out of his cock, practically blinding me. The other man orders him to untie me and pulls me off *the bed and to my knees. He squeezes my arm hard and twists it behind my back as the guy who brought me in there positions himself in front of me, his cock glistening with cum and jerking in excited anticipation. He threatens me, saying if I hurt him, scratch his cock in any way with my teeth, I'll be sorry. I hold his cock with my hand and slowly take it into my mouth. It's bitter with semen at the end of it. I'm on my knees with the other guy behind me pounding my ass and spanking me while calling me things like a "fucking pussy whore." The penis in my mouth swells even more as I gag. His semen cums spurting out against my throat, and I swallow, coughing and crying. The man fucking me from behind holds my head, banging it against the dresser as he shoots his cum into my ass. The pain is so great, I end up passing out. When I awake, they're all gone.*

In our fantasies, the elaborately described use of force frees us to experience whatever sexual variations we desire. It's worrisome—to put it mildly—that some of us use the "rape" word when, indeed, what almost always is sought is freedom from responsibility.

In past interviews with psychoanalysts and therapists, it's been noted that the "attacker" in the fantasy often stands for the incestuously desired father or brother. And while some women and men note that they have actually had sexual interludes with fathers or brothers, others acknowledge that it is only in fantasy that they are forced into sex by a powerful male figure, who was originally desired in childhood.

In the masochistically experienced sexual act in fantasy, we can permit ourselves to satisfy our desire for sexual pleasure and at the same time expiate the guilt.

Fauzia

Fauzia, a nineteen-year-old Pakistani woman who is a virgin, recounts a time at a friend's house when she was watching a movie.

A guy sitting next to me on the couch tried to get me to drink alcohol, which is forbidden in Islam, and to walk me home. I declined, but for some strange reason, I love to fantasize about him when I masturbate. I imagine he walks me to my dorm, then he asks if he can come inside to use the bathroom. I allow him in, but as soon as he's inside, he kisses me. He slips his hand under my shirt and cups my breasts. He squeezes them and pinches my nipples. He pushes me down on the bed and removes my shirt. He licks my nipples then starts to nurse, licking so hard they become sore. My clitoris starts to throb. He removes my panties and rubs my pussy really hard. I cry out in pain, and I know he has gone too far. "Stop!" I scream. He pins me down with the weight of his own body. He sticks the tip of his enormous penis in my vagina but has difficulty getting in all the way because of my hymen. He thrusts very hard to get inside me. "You're hurting me!" I cry, my voice drowned out by the vigorous squeaking of the mattress. He doesn't pay attention and grunts, "Tight hot pussy!" He fucks me so hard I can feel him ramming my cervix. I stop crying and love his hot dick fucking my pussy. My feet are far above my head. He doesn't care though. Then, we both climax, with his cum shooting into me.

In reality, I don't know why I fantasize this. I would never want it to happen. I don't even care about him. I think you can call what he did attempted rape. Furthermore, I believe sex and love should go together. I was never hit by my parents, so I don't believe I associate love with pain. When I fantasize about this creepy guy, however, I cum every time.

It is especially hard for women to separate sex and love. By confusing them, we risk losing the best of both. But for both men and women, though corporal punishment and sexual abuse may not be a necessity to planting the seeds of our S&M fantasies, what better way to nurture their growth?

Jeff

Jeff, a thirty-one-year-old professional, was abused by his father, who would whack him almost daily ten or twelve times with his belt.

The pain could not be described with words, but searing, burning, and unbearable come close. During the beatings, I was filled with rage but fearful of expressing anything other than tears. I also remember seeing my father naked after a bath and experiencing some sexual stirring as well as fear of his strength, power, and emotional distance. My mother also sexually and physically abused me. I have bodily memories of her fondling my testicles, moving them in her hand like two marbles. I believe she did this when she bathed me, and when she put me to sleep, she would lie down beside me and put her hand in my pajamas. She also gave me suppositories and enemas regularly at a very early age. She would call me into the toilet when she was changing her sanitary pad. She would tell me to bring her a clean one and hand me the dirty one, wrapped in toilet paper, to throw away.

I have a very good imagination and have had just about every type of sexual fantasy with people of almost every age and with both sexes. I have learned that fantasies, any fantasies, are OK. Most of my fantasies are about hurting women, embarrassing, controlling, and humiliating them. Making them submit to my will, making them powerless. Spanking them. Pushing my penis into their rectum, giving them douches with vinegar and soapy enemas, shaving their pubic hair. Sometimes, I pretend I am a woman. I fuck my ass with a hairbrush handle and spank myself imagining what a woman feels like when she is getting fucked. My best orgasms come from anal stimulation. I fantasize a man raping me. Sometimes, I fantasize about sucking a man's cock. Mouthing it when it is soft, making it hard, making it explode in my mouth, and swallowing the sperm. I also think about putting my penis in a submissive man that I just spanked or otherwise humiliated. I am intensely attracted to women but also filled with anger toward them. I am afraid of men and probably afraid of my sexual feelings toward them. People should realize that when they hit their children on the buttocks, they are sexually stimulating them. Don't hit your children. There are better ways to discipline them.

If I pinch or bite you, and you have an enlarged pleasure range, you may not experience it as pain. That is real life. In fantasy, we control the pain to the degree we desire, within our limits of pleasure. In reality, masochists often cannot control the pleasure range of pain and end up getting hurt. Some people in our society label consenting adults as perverts because they enjoy a certain amount of pain in sex. Sadder still, they condemn themselves for simply *thinking* sexually masochistic thoughts that arouse them.

Condemnation for our fantasies is a sad waste. The thought is not the deed! Given the cruelty of our real world nowadays and the breakdown of societal rules, especially in the home, where our sexual identity is formed, are we surprised that our sexual fantasies and real lives have become dramatically more permissive than ever before? Is it good/is it bad isn't the point.

What matters isn't societal condemnation of what turns us on sexually—but the finger-wagging, overbearing conscience within each of us that is usually far more brutal.

THE VICARIOUS RAPE FANTASY, OR,
"I'm Impervious to Pain—Except My Own"

"Find the pleasure through the pain," the fantasy man who has enslaved her says. As often as not, it's the threat of punishment rather than actual pain that brings on orgasm. Just as the threat of discovery heightens the thrill when we are stealing sex with an illicit partner.

Seth

Seth, a forty-three-year-old male teacher and PhD, happily married for twenty years, says his wife lost interest in sex when she had children, but recently, her drive resurfaced.

He divides his fantasies. When he is having sex with his wife, he employs a variety of other fantasies, saving for masturbation his fantasies of his wife being gang-raped while he watches. I find it interesting because it shows how masturbation can be an outlet for one aspect of our sexuality, and intercourse involves a reality-fantasy in tune with our partner.

I have a lot of fantasies. Sometimes, my wife and I "exchange" fantasies. One I got when a friend told me how he, walking with his wife in a very lonesome place, was suddenly surrounded by four young men on motorbikes, who taunted him by telling him his wife was ugly. I imagined this happening to us. It's not an accident that I use this fantasy when my wife and I have had a quarrel that has not been resolved.

Whether my wife is beautiful or not, they rape her in front of me; one in her cunt, one in her ass, one in her mouth, and the fourth she has to masturbate. Sometimes, I imagine my being forced to undress her and to clean their penises after they have fucked my wife. This fantasy is a strange mixture of sadistic and masochistic elements. I am a little ashamed of the sadistic fantasies but very much ashamed about the masochistic fantasies because "men have to be strong" and that kind of stuff.

Patricia

Patricia is a university-educated young woman in her twenties, who describes her-self as coming from a middle-class background with no "religious strings." She grew up in Europe and has traveled a lot. She says her fantasies are a mixture of things she actually did, would like to do, and some she never wants to do. In the ones she never wants to do, she watches as a third person, deriving a vicarious pleasure.

It's strange because if I feel pain during real sex, I can't have an orgasm, but while fantasizing about pain, I can. Presently, my fantasies are centered around this absolutely crazy guy I met some months back. I thought I knew my body and what I liked, but he definitely showed me my deficits! I'd never met a man who could get me this aroused in three seconds flat. I was so dripping wet and hot. I think I actually bit him because I couldn't get that lovely fat cock inside me fast enough—and in my fantasy, that's exactly what he's doing—fucking me wherever we might be at that moment, like maybe on a kitchen table.

In other fantasies, the participants are kind of faceless; in any case, not people I know. I don't enter these fantasies as myself. For a few seconds, I might take the role of either man or woman, but mostly, I'm kind of a distant watcher. My present fantasy is about a young woman who has been kidnapped. She doesn't remember anything but comes to in a strange room, naked and tied spread-eagled on a bed. A few minutes later, a man walks in, quite good-looking, naked, and with an enormous cock already hard as a rock. He calmly tells her he's going to fuck her. She struggles and begs him not to. But he just laughs, spreads her, and pushes his prick into her. She screams because he is thrusting hard and deep. After a while, her screams turn to sobs as she realizes she can't fight him. When she thinks it's over, he just changes her position and says, "I want you from behind." He has various instruments in the cupboard nearby, like cushions to place under her and sashes and leather cuffs to hold her in place. He ties her up loosely and goes to work.

In the weeks that follow, he introduces various sexual toys, all made of cold metal, which are designed to spread her and increase her pain. Sometimes, the man fucks her mouth or invites a friend (usually black, if the first one is white), and they both fuck her. He also has a collection of videos of similar activities, so he can watch them while he fucks the woman and keep it up longer.

Even before I knew what a cock was, I had fantasies along these lines.

So much is laid down in the first years when we were soft as clay. But dependency is not always pleasant. Nowhere are we more at odds with Mother than in matters surrounding our genitals, that area that is so instrumental in sexual pleasure. We learn to hold our bladder and bowels and either abandon altogether touching our genitals—except to wipe ourselves clean—or we do it in secret. Before we've even found a partner in the crime of sexual pleasure, we have so woven the spice of "forbidden" into touching ourselves, stealth and near discovery are laced into not just the act of sexual feeling but also the thought.

Without bidding the fantasy to appear, our minds go to the images that accelerate the first flame of eros. We are held and kissed, maybe just a handhold, and the circuitry ignites the home movies in our head that never fail.

That so many of us, male and female, climb to orgasm on images of restraint, imminent terror, and punishment speaks of the longevity of life's earliest lessons regarding our bodies. No one wants to think that a child is taking in the basic lessons of later sexual feeling. Were you raised to respect, admire, and care for that place between your legs? Of course, the climb to orgasm has to get past the early denials and obstacles laid down when we were too young to know that we were being programmed.

FANTASIES OF CASTRATION, OR,
"My Testicles Are Your Testicles"

Nick

I'm a twenty-three-year-old with two basic fantasies—one of them about dominance and the other submission. I think of submission more and more.

My fantasy of submission involves a woman in her mid-thirties to early forties. Her women friends are at her house, and she is going to give them a show. I am nude on my knees with my face down on the bed, with my ass in the air and my legs spread. My fantasy woman is wearing something sexy and comes from behind and starts stroking my hard cock and pulling it back between my legs. She sucks my balls, first one, then the other. She sticks her finger in my ass while she strokes my cock. Her friends look on.

She usually ends it by jacking me off so my cum shoots into her hand, and she spreads it all over my ass. Sometimes, she takes out one of those large kitchen knives and presses the flat of the blade against my ass and balls so I can feel the coldness of it. Then, she firmly grabs my ball sac in one hand and puts the dull edge of the blade against my scrotum and tells me she could "Cut my fucking nuts off." This is to show her power.

Dominic

A young man in his late twenties, Dominic has an innocent face and a nice smile. He's a blue-collar guy who sees himself as rugged and virile.

I've had a lot of girls. I'm always sexually attracted to "take charge" types. My fantasy involves my being the possession of a very beautiful, strong, confident woman. She's dominant and classy. We live in a spacious contemporary home, which is always immaculate. My duties include cleaning the house, making meals, washing clothes, and giving massages to my "owner." When she is really tense, I sit on the floor and give her oral, anal, and vaginal massages. One day, she comes home raging mad because I have cheated on her with a neighbor. To put me in my place, she has my testicles removed surgically. This gives her much delight.

When the surgery is over, she has me wear short skirts around the house. She has me dress totally as a woman, complete with bra and wig. When she gives a party at her house, she has me raise my miniskirt to show the women "what happens to naughty boys."

Joshua

Joshua is a thirty-five-year-old blue-collar worker in the Bible belt. He had a good marriage for two years until his mother-in-law started a rumor that he was having an affair with someone at work.

We went for a year without having sex. Then, when my wife found out I was masturbating, she got mad and made me move out. My first fantasies started when I was fifteen and began masturbating. Much to my mortification at the time, my first fantasy involved my mother. Looking back on it now, I realize it was probably because she was the only woman I had ever seen nude at that point in my life. I soon learned to fantasize about girls I knew. That was a great relief.

The next noteworthy fantasy involved asking a girlfriend to put a diaper on me and fill it with mashed potatoes, then scold me for messing my diaper. She would fondle me while cleaning me up. Another fantasy involved having sex with me and my partner wearing one big messy diaper.

Once my marriage was on the rocks and sex was on the decline, I started masturbating more frequently about the women I saw online. My favorite to date is to be tied to the bed and teased, to be kept for hours at a time erect without an orgasm. In between teasing me, she will sit on my face and force me to perform oral sex. The force isn't necessary, since I love oral sex anyway. But I enjoy being shown I'm not in control. She will have three or four orgasms in this manner before allowing me to have one. Then, when she decides it's time for my reward, she performs oral sex on me while using a vibrator in my anus and rubbing her vagina all over my face.

I also have a similar fantasy in which I visit a sadistic mistress wearing a pair of pink panties. I imagine she ties a wire around my testicles, with the other end tied to a door, just to see how much torture I will withstand in order to please her. When she gets mad because I cry too much, she slams the door, slicing off my testicles.

We live in a world of stress, competition, real and imagined danger. Nothing can be counted on to stay in place, not just in our physical world but in the world of intangibles: fidelity, honesty, trust, and, oh yes, love ongoing.

But we can control ourselves and to a degree, if we are clever, the people around us. We decide not to fall in love, not to depend on or trust anyone; people let you down, betray you. Their word means nothing. Who needs them? We lock ourselves up and throw away the key. Now no one can get at us. After a while, no one tries.

So much for love. What about sex? The tricky bit about sex is that when it's good, really good, many of us fall in love. We didn't mean to, but he or she is there, in our minds, making us weak and needy. Afterward, we lie on the sofa, dreaming, replaying again and again what it felt like in our beloved's arms the night before. In these dreamy recreations, we can't resist putting our hand between our legs, closing our eyes, and awaiting once again the climb to orgasm. But we are rigid, our minds still on work left at the office. How to let go? Fantasies of force *make us* give up the iron restraints as someone more powerful than we *demands* we let go: "Beyond my control!"

Bruce, with a degree in physics and an MBA, says, "When the woman takes the initiative, it feels like permission for me to enjoy myself or when I'm forced to have sex, that also heightens the orgasm. In my relationships with women, I have sometimes found it difficult to 'let go' and fully enjoy myself and gain pleasure. I think this affects my fantasies, as they seem to revolve around situations where I am explicitly given 'permission' to enjoy myself or am 'forced to enjoy myself.'"

MEN AND THE WOMEN WHO RAPE THEM, OR,
"What's a Nice Girl Like You Doing with Handcuffs and a Dildo Like That?"

Teddy

Teddy, a young man with a master's degree and a job in desktop publishing, says he too loves women who are supremely confident. He fantasizes becoming a beautiful woman's slave.

She has many female lovers. Though I know she enjoys men as well, I never see them. The other women in the house are younger. They all enjoy abusing me. Slapping me, sodomizing me with their dildos. One of my mistress's nieces, eighteen years old, straps on a dildo and fucks me up the ass for hours. I cry out, as the pain is excruciating. But my mistress barely notices.

Logan

Logan is an industrialist, happily married, with two beautiful daughters. His dad was a small-town psychiatrist. His mother was very strict, and sex was a forbidden topic in the house. I find it interesting that he uses his uncle's new wife for his discipline fantasy, the seeds of which were undoubtedly planted by his mother.

We four brothers and three sisters were always afraid of our mother's anger. When I was quite young and innocent regarding sex, I was sodomized by an elder cousin who fooled me into believing that taking his cock up my ass would build my muscles. I was dying to be a bodybuilder gymnast then.

At about the same time, my uncle married a beautiful buxom woman. I was so aroused by her big tits that I used to steal her 38D cup bra from her bedroom. I would sniff the perfume mixed with her sweat. I would madly kiss her bra, then masturbate on it. The aroma of her worn panties drove me to dizzy heights. Sometimes, I used to wear her bra and panties. That gave me the strongest erections.

In my fantasy, she finds me in her room with her bra. She decides to spank me in order to correct me. The sound of her glass bangles as she spanks me is music to my ears. The pain turns to pleasure. The spanking is so erotic that I can't help myself and cum on her petticoat. The cum soaks through her petticoat onto her thighs. She gets angry and orders me to lick her clean. She pulls me by my hair and pushes me into her soaking wet crotch of her black nylon panties. I am also ordered to lick her asshole. I part her buttocks, inhaling the sweet aroma of her rosebud anus. She puts a dog collar and a leash on my neck and pulls me to her four-poster bed. She lies facedown on the bed and puts a pillow under her pelvis so that her milk-white, luscious buttocks are raised high in the air. "Come, slave. Lick your mistress's ass," is her command. I usually cum at this point in my fantasy.

Forrest

Forrest is a Southern lawyer in his thirties who still finds his wife extremely beautiful. It's interesting that in times of stress, his desire to be dominated increases.

My mother was strict, and my fantasies have always concerned the same general topic: female domination. My sex life with others has always been heterosexual, usually in the realm of the normal as opposed to the kinky. However, I have noticed that during periods of stress, my desire for the kinky increases, wanting to completely turn my will over to a powerful woman. During the last year, my wife and I have begun exploring dominant and submissive sexual relations with largely good results. Last summer, she announced to me that she was interested in watching some adult videos. I rented movies I knew contained scenes which dovetailed with my sexual desires. As we watched the movies, she announced that she wanted to fuck me up the ass with a strap-on dildo. It spawned this fantasy:

I come home from work, and a hostile look appears on her face. "You want supper?" she asks. "Why, yes, honey, I do," I respond. "Well, motherfucker, I have had about enough of taking orders from you. Things are going to be different tonight."

She attaches a set of handcuffs to me, slings me down on the bed, and I look up at her as she removes her gown to reveal a black leather outfit. She is wearing a bra-like thing with no real cups but merely studded straps which encircle her breasts. "What has gotten into you, baby?" I ask. She stuffs a phallic-shaped gag in my mouth. Then, she walks back to her dresser and picks up a cat-o'-nine tails. "Stand up," she orders. The first blow from the cat on my back is vicious. The steel from the handcuffs bites into my flesh. She proceeds to cut my boxers off. She grabs my rock-hard dick and says, "What would you do if I had one of these? And told you I was going to butt-fuck you with it." She looks me in the eye with an amused, slightly sinister look on her face. I shrug.

She goes to the dresser, pulls out a large curved dildo, and I scream in agony as she sodomizes me with it.

I love this feeling of being violated. Of feeling an object in my ass and knowing that there is a beautiful woman on the other end of it.

I relayed this fantasy, and we tried it. She followed my fantasy as I had described it to her—to a "T." It hurt like a motherfucker. If "May your fantasies come true" is not an old gypsy curse, it ought to be. I discovered quickly I am not a masochist. She really got into it though. Needless to say, after it was over, I suggested we rethink this fantasy business.

I believe there is no trip like orgasm, nothing comparable. For a few moments, we are outside our skin, flying, floating, our mind cleared of all the obligatory facts of life. There is that moment before we let go when we know it's going to happen, a most precious, incomparable moment. We wonder why we waited so long to take this journey. But "be careful what you wish for." As Forrest shows, fantasy is ruled by a very different set of laws than reality, where it helps to understand and honor our physical limitations.

FEMALE SADISTIC FANTASIES, OR,
"Don't Get Mad—Get Even"

Women come in all shades of anger these days, all degrees of toughness. In my own little world, I'd say the women I know are as quick to anger, faster on the draw, and can be more vengeful than men when crossed.

The dark side of women was there before, simply camouflaged by practiced girlish denials: "Hate her? Of course not. We love her!" With fewer chips to play with, our ammo back then was emotional withdrawal from the victim, the withholding of our love, as in, "Give her the treatment!" Meaning, "Don't ask that pretty girl to the party." Today, we play with the same chips as men but still cling to our traditional revenge, the tried and true, when one of "our group" gets more than her share of the pie.

Once upon a time, men looked forward to well-behaved children, dinner, and a smiling wife and, maybe later that night, sex, though the marital deal didn't promise the kind of sex men once dreamed of. Many men didn't see their wives in that role nor did the women once they became mothers. For great sex, dirty sex, men went to bad girls.

Perhaps politicians, such as Eliot Spitzer, whose careers are based on a persona of respectability, advocating virtue and decency, are living closer to a world of forty years ago. It's very telling that Spitzer, with so much to lose, was willing to risk his career in order to fulfill his sexual needs.

Obviously, there was a reason that men deprived themselves of a mate who had an erotic engine of her own. How could he hold his head high, putting his shoulder to the wheel of industry, if his mind was preoccupied with fantasies of his wife having it off with every other man she encountered? Better to neuter the wife and find great sex with bad girls.

Sometimes, I feel like Methuselah, reminding those of you who weren't around prior to feminism what it was like before the world changed. There was a lot at stake keeping women out of touch with our influence, given that we raised the human race. We simply didn't think of it that way. And when we did, the world changed. It happened overnight. A tiny spark caught fire, and women became the powerful force we are today. Once put in a position of competing with men—and other women—for the job, we got off that pedestal so fast it was dizzying. I imagine even Doris Day, now a single entrepreneur, happily gave up the Doris Day persona.

Once we could pay the rent and put food on the table, the rigid rules that had defined what a woman was were rewritten. We were anything a man could be, including aggressive, vindictive, mean, and, yes, killers. The fantasies that we swore we didn't have were now available. We could say, "Oh, I understand wanting to tie someone up, climb on top of him, and..."

During the Iraq war, well-known photos of a female soldier physically abusing an Iraqi prisoner, all the while smoking a cigarette and posing for the camera, sent shivers around the world. But no one suggested that it was a fake. No one said a woman couldn't possibly do such a thing. We no longer deny women's power or dark side. We know they can possess man's capability for cruelty. Nor do we argue the correctness of men raising children as women go to war.

The women in this book have a field day punishing men in erotic fantasies of sadomasochism, as lurid as any invented by men in the past. Reading their fantasies, one can't help wondering where this killer creativity used to go in the distant days of "women, the caring, loving sex."

When reading Ursula's email, my first inclination was to put it aside as too extreme. I told myself, "Stop editing what doesn't appeal to you." The more brutal this woman's fantasy, the more aroused she gets. She has fantasies of raping men and has been raped herself. She is furious at men for having raped her in reality and says, "My fantasies are brutal, but they help me have an orgasm." The tone of these young women when describing the giving or getting of brutal punishment unsettles me. Did I miss something? I go back and reread. All the brutality, real and fantasy, there it is in black and white, no tricks, no pretend. This is how it is.

Ursula

When I was eighteen, I was raped in a city park by a boy I'd only met a few days before. A few years later, I met an older man who made me feel like the most important person in the world. Our lovemaking was gentle and satisfying, until about three years into the relationship, when he started sticking objects in my vagina that really hurt. It's like he started thinking of me as an object and wasn't concerned about my needs anymore. What he did felt more like torture than love. So I left.

I started becoming very angry with men. I was told that women's sexual needs were as important as men's, so I decided to use men the way they had used me. This started a four-year behavior in search of sexual satisfaction and power. I think some men realized I was using them, and I got raped several times—once gang-raped. After that, I was even angrier because I felt like they were using their penises like weapons against women. I started having fantasies about raping men. I knew women could rape men even though I had been told it was impossible. It doesn't take a genius to know you can drug a guy, tie him up, and ram a dildo up his ass. You can also force him at gunpoint to do anything you want orally.

Sometimes, my fantasies are brutal, but they help me have an orgasm when I masturbate. In college, on an anonymous questionnaire, they asked us if we ever fantasized about rape. When I answered "Yes," I was wondering how they would know if my fantasies were of raping or being raped.

Even before I started looking at porn, I was having fantasies about raping men. I was very aroused by women overpowering men. Usually, I would tie them up, beat them, and rape them. The more brutal the fantasy, the more aroused I would become, and the better the orgasm. I even found a website where women were actually killing men. I guess you can tell that I'm pretty frustrated with men and the sexual inequalities in our society.

We're taught that killing is a sin, too emotionally traumatic to ever fully get over. Why would the serial killer commit such horrific acts of violence? But many serial killers are driven by a sexual need, says Dr. Laurence Tancredi. "There is even a case of a woman who may have escaped the death sentence had she not confessed that during the killing she orgasmed."

Claudette

Obese and hypertensive due to abuse in her childhood, Claudette had her first date at twenty-two. She says her mother was "an expert at psychosomatic illnesses."

In my fantasy, I am eighteen and in a futuristic society. I work in a residence kitchen, and after work, I am delivered to a suite and chained to a wall. Shortly after, an older professional man enters. He says he is a "sexual initiator." He does his job with finesse, and we continue our relationship until I become hugely pregnant. In another, I choose to work as an official prostitute for an order of monks. (Maybe this can be explained in part by a twenty-year friendship with a monk with heretical inclinations.) The rule is that they cannot be virgins before they join the order. I am responsible for certifying they have performed full heterosexual intercourse before the initiation. Some of the ways the initiation involving mutilation and restraint is done include self-amputation of the penis and scrotum with a cheese wire, by piranha fish, by surgery (with or without anesthesia), or by being sewn into a horsehair g-string. I am also responsible for the sexual rehabilitation of former inmates (who did not join the order voluntarily).

Margaret

Margaret, who grew up in a small Midwestern town, shares words as mean as anything I've heard from men. For that reason, I include her letter, though I've never doubted the fairer sex's appetite for cruelty.

I have been suppressing my sadistic desires for years and trying to be a good female like I've been told. I just can't do it anymore. You probably won't print anything as brutal as this.

But my mom was brutal. I was physically abused by her growing up. She could be very nice sometimes and very mean other times. My first sexual experiences were with my brother, who is several years younger than me. When I was about twelve, I tied him up and had sex with him. I'm twenty-three now and have been raped several times. I am very angry with men because they always seem to have more sexual freedom than women. Women always seem to be victims, and it is "normal" for men to want to hurt women and be sadistic.

Because women are supposed to be "the good ones," I've been suppressing my sadistic side for years. I just can't do it anymore. If a man is sadistic, he is "normal"; a sadistic woman is a pervert.

I have a fantasy where a man is trying to rape me, but I put him in his place. I manage to surprise him and turn him so he's on the bottom and I'm on top. I take out my gun and put it to his throat. I then cuff his hands. I tell him he is to cooperate or I will kill him. I love to see a man bleed. I take out my knife and cut him, and he screams in pain. I put the knife to his penis and tell him to be quiet or I'll cut it off. After I fuck him, I no longer need him. I tell him that I have lied and have decided to kill him anyway. I cut his throat until the life is out of him. Now all I have to do is discard the rest of the male population in this way.

At the end of the day, I come back to reread Margaret's words. Surely these fantasies of anger at men must have had conscious or subconscious existence among women when life was more restricting under patriarchy. If you were an adventurous, assertive woman, didn't swallowing all that make you full of rage? But "nice girls" didn't feel killer resentments, so neither did we. Like our sexual fantasies, we made them disappear.

One thing is clear in these more recent fantasies: women have become aware of the power that they own as women. Elise says, "Being able to take the initiative feels like permission for me to enjoy myself."

I've fought for feminism, marched for it, and became a writer of books because of it. But every revolution has its downside, the unavoidable side effects of any great enterprise that turns the world upside down. And we women really did dismantle patriarchy by moving out of the home and into the workplace.

It was a grand revolution, the opportunity for half of the human race to define themselves as something other than mother and housekeeper. Not that the role, God knows, was without value. The person who raises the human race—feeds, comforts, and disciplines—is forming the next generation. Most men were shadow-figures to their children under patriarchy, which wasn't good for either man or child. Only when it got really bad was the discipline that was generally laid down by mother handed over with a stern "Wait till your father gets home!"

But under patriarchy, we did have a world of clear right and wrong. It was drummed into us as small children until it became who and how we were. When we broke the rules, which we often did, we knew we had erred. We felt something called guilt.

As the Internet pats a reassuring hand, we find less guilt in either the fantasies or the real lives of people today. Sometimes, a man or woman will bring up the guilty feeling as a booster to the erotic thrill experienced in, say, a fantasy of sex with the best friend's spouse.

Today, with less flavoring from the salt and peppering of guilt, erotic fantasies reach for more charged scenes, imaginary and lived out—scenes that were unspoken in the past, as in incest and a rainbow of S&M.

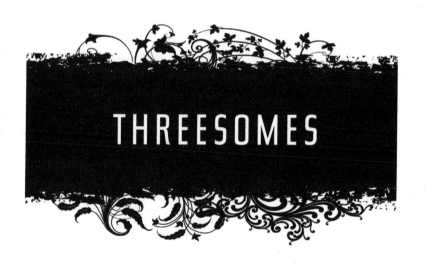

THREESOMES

THREESOMES

The need for more: I remember my first threesome—and almost my last. It was a day in spring. The birds were chirping, the squirrels and woodland animals of New York City were playing, and I was full of optimism. I'd just met this fascinating man, tall, attractive, full of wit, knowledgeable about everything, and, clearly, quite taken with me. And it wasn't as though I didn't have other men whom I was also seeing/bedding/semi-in-love with. So, when it transpired one sunny May day that he and I and this other charming fellow were lunching at a Chinese restaurant and the heat between the three of us built to a temperature demanding relief, the two of them led me to bed. No, wait, let's be honest: always the leader, I picked up their intent and merrily took them both in hand to bed.

All in a blink, the sun clouded over, the birds shut up, and I smelled a rat: jealousy, envy, and that old left-out feeling that was rooted in my earliest days. Oh, damn, shit—I was merely a conduit in these two men's fantasies. Neither had had sex with a man before, but the fantasy was clearly there. A jealous person can smell that old "third wheel feeling" a mile away.

I pulled it off. No one was going to see me diminished. I went through a little hell that afternoon, performing like an erotic acrobat, even bringing the two of them to cum together. And then I dressed, bid them a merry "Hi-ho! It's-been-great-guys!" goodbye. And walked up Fifth Avenue, casting neither a shadow nor a reflection in the windows of Bergdorf Goodman.

Let me add that if I hadn't cared deeply for one of these men, the tale would be different, as indeed it was a few years later when I enjoyed a three-way with two men who were friends and nothing more. Now, here is my confession. I did it not just out of lust but to test myself, to prove what I had always sensed. That, for me, a threesome is not something that can be hastily entered into.

Don't let me diminish the ecstasy so many of you find in a threesome. We are all different. Our different pasts and biology trigger different levels of emotions, but given jealousy's deep roots, think about your fantasy of you and your beloved and a third party and weigh the pleasure principle carefully.

Need I remind you that this scene works brilliantly for many. Certainly, in fantasy, a threesome is something to be run and rerun again through all its combinations and permutations. This erotic ballet sometimes performs best with near strangers. If it's voyeurism that gets you hot, watch the two of them go at it. If you are the erotic acrobat, feel the stimulation, the fantasy of them watching you. It is about the three of you playing off one another. What more can you ask?

TAKE MY HUSBAND—PLEASE!

Interestingly, there are those of us who are rigid in our desire not to live out our erotic dreams and others who anticipate breathing life into them. With regard to the latter, I imagine it takes a strong sense of self. Maybe you can handle the variations and permutations of a threesome. For Natasha and her first husband, it was a voyeur's/exhibitionist's paradise.

Natasha

A middle-aged woman who lost her first husband in a car crash, Natasha has now been married to another wonderful man for four years.

I'm an advertising and marketing manager for a mid-sized communications company. I had a comfortable childhood in a very upper-middle-class suburb in the Midwest and was a virgin when I married my first husband. But I knew I wanted to try everything. There was one particularly ribald sexual evening in New York when I was first married. We went to a swing club. At first, we simply watched the other couples, but we finally overcame our timidity and joined in. I'll never forget the excitement of watching Morris being sucked by two women while their husbands sucked and fucked me to climax after climax. At one point, I looked over to see one of the women on top of my husband, fucking him, while the other sat on his face while he sucked her. Even when we were back in our hotel room, sated at three in the morning, I couldn't resist teasing Morris's red, wilted prick with my tongue until he became hard again. He fucked me until daybreak while we talked about the couples we had met at the club.

About two years after Morris's death, something happened that awakened the sexual juices in me. It was near midnight on a Friday night, and I heard noises. I got up and peered down the stairs and was about to call out when I realized it was my son, Jeremy, naked except for his boxer shorts, pulling down the panties of a young girl. She was sitting on the edge of the couch, and as he jerked the panties off her feet, she put them on the edge of the couch and pushed her legs wide open. Jeremy bent down and began kissing her cunt while she ran her fingers through his hair.

Myriad emotions ran through me. I wanted to yell out for them to stop. Yet, I was fascinated watching the slim young girl rock back and forth and whisper to my son as he licked her. Then, Jeremy stood up, and the girl frantically pulled his shorts down. I gasped. His prick looked huge in the half-light. She smiled up at him and began to suck him. He lunged forward, fucking her mouth. I felt my hand stroking my cunt. I was ashamed but couldn't help myself.

THE TRADITIONAL: MALE FANTASIES OF TWO WOMEN
"Imagine Me and You and You"

Even in fantasy, another person satisfying my lover can leave me cold and, yes, a little sad. But for many, like Richard, the thought of being with two women can bring soaring highs.

Richard

Richard, a twenty-eight-year-old white male, nonpracticing Catholic, says he and his wife, Gwen, have a solid marriage and can talk about anything and everything.

I remember one day, in my early fantasy life, I found this picture of two women together. They were beautiful and sexy, and I was fascinated by them. That became my main sexual fantasy, and it remains my number one today. I've even made it come to pass a few times, much to everyone's delight.

This is one of my favorites. This one almost happened, so that is why I like it so much. It has to do with the babysitter we hired just after our daughter was born, a sophomore at the university studying to be a nurse. In the fantasy, I tell her about our past threesome experiences.

She asks questions and then I tell her Gwen and I think that she is very attractive and that we would like her to join us. The talk gets hot, and Gwen says she is getting turned on. Bett, the babysitter, then goes over to Gwen and kisses her lightly on the lips and tells her that she is very pretty and she would like to have sex with her. Gwen responds to her, and they kiss and slowly undress each other.

Bett wants to eat Gwen first. Gwen complies and then Bett begins to lick her slowly, something Gwen loves. She encircles her clit and then comes down the other side of her pussy. She is driving Gwen wild. I am naked, jerking off to the whole scene. Gwen goes wild and has her first orgasm. She tells Bett that she wants to repay her. She goes in for her first taste of pussy and takes a few small licks. She likes her taste and begins lapping faster. This drives Bett wild, and she cums all over Gwen's face. Then, Bett sees me and tells me that it has been awhile since she had a dick and would I help her out? I say sure, so I begin to fuck her while Gwen cradles her in her arms and kisses and caresses her tits.

MAKING THE FANTASY A REALITY

I've watched the secretive threesome transform into the easily accessible common-day pleasure available to anyone with a will and Internet provider. A friend may now mention, with a certain blush, the incredible night she had with two men, two women, a man and a woman, and our mind soars; excitement, lust, we feel closer to her or we feel jealousy, envy, denial. Some of us want to know more. How/where do we get the tickets for this ride? The real question is, from the daunting amount of options online, how do we choose?

As my gay friend Michael says, "It's like a fine wine—you just have to try them all." Interspersed throughout this chapter are some of the ads quickly found from online personal sites, such as Craigslist, posted to make fantasy a reality.

Seeking My Last First Date – 47

Looking for My Last First Date. A special ladies to Hold, Kiss, Love & Fall Asleep, wrapped around each other. I am a very down to earth, good looking (so I have been told) guy who believes that ROMANCE IS NOT DEAD, it's just taken somewhat of a beating lately. I am a very romantic, caring, sensitive, compassionate man, with a great sense of humor & smile, interested in meeting two very open minded ladies who understands the true meaning of romance & commitment. I love hugging & kissing, music, dancing & making the two of you feel like you are the only ones in this big world. I also love the outdoors, anything to do with the water, nature, kids. I enjoy going to the clubs from time to time. I also love candle lit dinners with soft music in the background, whether out or at home (I enjoy cooking, I am a very good cook), while holding hands, hugging, kissing, dancing & I enjoy those moments we share at home just the three of us. I am looking for a two beautiful ladies for a committed relationship, which would include romance, flowers & all of the above, forever. I am not a 1 woman man. I have been described as "A really sweet guy", "A Big Mush", & someone that seems "Too good to be true". Am I "Mr. Wonderful"? Not by a long shot, but I am a "Really Sweet Guy", that wants to share his life with a "two really Sweet Ladies". I am looking for those 2 special women that I can kiss goodnight & then kiss good morning. We can walk hand in hand through whatever life puts in front of us. We have all seen elderly couples holding hands; well I don't want to be one of them. The ladies I would love to meet, would be pretty outside & gorgeous inside. Two women that will be themself & knows what they wants from a man & a relationship. Believes that "Trust, honesty, mutual respect, communication, open minded & a great sense of humor" are necessary to make a relationship work. Two ladies with a kind heart that wants to share it with that 1 special man, enjoys being spoiled & pampered, but not smothered, & is looking for a handsome, very romantic, affectionate, sensual man. Most importantly, two women that are ready to start the next phase of her life with "New Luggage" instead of "Old Baggage". This is my wish list. Am I living in a fantasy, the romantic hopes not. Please respond with a description of yourself & what you are looking for in a relationship, & a picture please, & I will immediately respond with a pic & phone #. Hope to hear from you soon.

Would You Like A Great Relationship While Also Being Promiscuous? — 48

I am looking for a very normal, healthy, fun, "conventional" type relationship when it comes to matters other than sex: Movies, concerts, DVDs, TV, listening to music, snuggling, conversation, exploring NYC, breakfast in bed, museums, theater, cooking together, romance—all of the good stuff that brings couples closer together. I crave and want that in my life again.

HOWEVER, I am also seeking a VERY sexually adventurous lifestyle with the right woman. I have been a swinger for most of my life (I'll be more specific below) and have dabbled in various kinks and scenes throughout the years. I want to continue in "the lifestyle" and find that women who are not into any of these things just don't do it for me sexually. I love women who are promiscuous, kinky and sexually adventurous—and who could pull that off within the confines of an otherwise "normal" and loving relationship.

As a swinger, I particularly enjoy threesomes and moresomes. I particularly enjoy sharing a hot woman in MFM threesomes and would also like someone to go to swing clubs and events with as well as hosting our own threesomes and moresomes at my place. Understand that this is not a sneaky way of me trying to get two women into bed. Been there, done that and, while I would certainly do that again, I think it is far hotter sharing my lady in a MFM threesome or moresome.

I have also enjoyed various kinks, role-play games, exhibitionism/voyeurism, discreet public "play," BDSM and other scenarios. None of these things are important fetishes to me, none are deal breakers, but they do open the door to some fun possibilities.

And when we are done being very naughty, we can curl up on the sofa to watch a fun DVD and tell each other bad jokes that somehow make us laugh anyway.

As for me, I am straight, 48, 5-10 tall, 200lbs, attractive, ethnic White, fun, easy-going, smart, educated. I have a warped sense of humor, can be quirky, quick witted and can be a smart ass at times.

As for you, any age is fine as long as our ages don't get in the way of us having a reasonable relationship. I like pretty girls—but that can mean many things. Primarily I go for a pretty face and women who dress and act like women (butch is out for me). Of course I like fit girls— but heavier girls are just fine if they carry it well and with confidence and feel & look pretty.

As for the lifestyle, I prefer to be with an experienced woman (experienced in the things

I mentioned above) with a definite naughty, slutty, promiscuous streak.

If what I've described sounds good to you please get in touch, tell me about yourself, what attracted you to my post and please send me a photo. I will send you mine as well. Any questions? Please ask away!

Larry

Larry, a writer, carries things a step farther and has three women, making it a foursome.

I am a male, thirty-three years old, and gregarious. I get along with people well. I have many fantasies but just one that I wish to share.

I work in a business environment where most of the females are not particularly attractive. Except one. Stephanie is my fantasy woman, and she occupies most of my fantasy time. She is about 5´5´´, 126 pounds, with dark eyes, jet-black, long, straight hair and the most round, perfect ass you could imagine. She and I have gotten to be good friends, but she has no clue as to my thoughts.

She is in charge of the computer system. In my fantasy, she calls me into her office to check out something on her screen. But that's not all I'm checking out! She is wearing a black V-neck top with Lycra pants. Her tits are almost visible through her blouse, and I can see the outline of her panties (pink!) through her pants. She leans over to get something, and I get a better glimpse of her tits. My dick gets hard. She senses I am turned on by her, and she suggests that we discuss the "computer problem" on Sunday when no one is around.

I take one look at her when I open the door Sunday, and I almost cum. She is in a tight miniskirt with a sexy blouse. Her gorgeous black hair looks great, and I can see that she too is yearning with desire.

Our mouths lock on each other, and our tongues begin to play. Meanwhile, her nipples are hard and pointy, and I slowly brush them with my fingers. She reaches down and feels my throbbing dick through my pants that I'm straining to remove.

I lick her neck as she arches her head back while she squeals in delight. She tongues my ears and begins to remove her clothes as quickly as possible.

I can't take it anymore, and I beg her to get on her knees to suck me off. She gets down, but she teases me by just lightly rubbing her moist tongue on the tip of my dick. I grab the back of her head and force my dick deep in her warm, loving, hot, saucy mouth.

But she gets up and begs me to fuck her deep inside. I just cream and cream the inside of her pussy after a long hot fuck session.

After we are all done, I realize that we are being watched through the window by two local teenage girls, who are clearly turned on. I invite them to join us, and with all three women at my feet, I am carried over the sky to another orgasm. This fantasy ends only to have the episode repeat itself next Sunday.

FEMALE FANTASIES OF TWO MEN
"Two Straight Men Are Hard to Find"

Perhaps I can more easily identify with the fantasy of one woman with two men, where I am the one clearly desired, a demanding order, with no guarantees. We jealous types prefer our threesomes in our favor. There are just too many bad memories from childhood for the likes of us, and (hard as they may be to find) two completely heterosexual males make for a perfect trio. Tread lightly while entering these waters, given that once you dive in, a real threesome is hard to get out of.

However, in fantasy, it's much easier to conjure up those 100% heterosexual males. A threesome in fantasy is a playground where both men and women enjoy scenes of multiple sex partners giving them all the pleasure hard to find with just one partner.

Patsy

I am nineteen years old from Texas and have had two intimate relationships. I love loud sex. I also like to be talked to "dirty" when I have sex, and I love to hear a guy talk about my body.

I have a lot of fantasies, but one of my favorites is the one where I'm a bimbo. You know the type, the cute cheerleaders who'll fuck anything, anytime, anywhere. I'm usually wearing a skirt, no panties, and a button-up shirt, no bra. I'm at a football game, and the home team has just lost, so I go down to the locker room to make the guys feel better. When I get there, there are only two guys left. One is the real athletic type, and the other is thinner, a kind of nerdy virgin.

I see the athletic one sitting on the bench with no shirt. He's a little dirty and sweaty from the game. He tells me to sit down on top of him. I do. He then starts to run his hands up my legs and under my skirt. Then, a smile starts across his face because he's found bare butt. I slide down a little so I can undo his pants and let out his now-erect cock. I then get on top of him and settle onto his large cock. By now my shirt is undone. He tells me to lean over so he can suck my tits.

It's now when I see the other guy. He's standing there holding his cock. It drives me crazy. I tell him to come over, and he does. I grab his cock and start sucking it. Then, the guys decide to turn me over so that I'm on my stomach on the bench with my ass in the air. One guy is behind me, and the other is in my mouth. We fuck until we all cum together.

Holly

I'm Holly, twenty-three, consider myself attractive, and since the age of five or six, my fantasies have had to do with threesomes and bondage. They range from elaborate scenarios to short images. I never fantasize about strangers, only about people I know and love. There is this one in which a friend of Leo's (my boyfriend) and mine (a really muscular, sexy, but very shy, guy) jokingly suggests we should all shower together. I would love to give this guy head with Leo looking on. Maybe even having Leo grab me by the hair on the back of my head forcing me down to suck the other guy's cock, forcing my head up and down while he nods his approval. Or sometimes, I gently kiss both of them in the shower as we all lather each other and then maybe hop into bed for a wonderful threesome.

Bobby

I'm a forty-seven-year-old widow, and in my fantasy, I pretend I'm having sex with two men, always being in control, making them fuck each other and suck each other off. Then, I switch back and forth from one cock to another until I make them both cum. Or sometimes, but not usually, another woman and I work over one man. We make him watch us 69 each other, suck each other's tits, kiss each other, and finally allow him to join in.

In reality, my husband died while we were having sex. He was my best friend, my lover, and my greatest playmate until his death at only thirty-seven years of age. He died making love to me on Christmas Eve of a massive heart attack; I still have not totally recovered from that horrible experience. I met him when I was only seventeen years old, and he was my first and only lover until death. I'm now alone. Believe me, I have heard every bad joke about dying in the saddle, a nightmare. If it weren't for masturbation, I would have no sex life at all.

Bobby's is a poignant story. Perhaps she finds comfort of a threesome in the insurance that if one should disappear, she wouldn't be alone again.

Elaine

Elaine, a college student and a virgin, always felt fat and ugly. Now she sees that perception as drawn out of insecurity. She also fantasizes having sex with two men. But one of the men is her obsession, a gay male friend. She watches him satisfied, top to bottom, by a male porn star before they both take care of her.

I consider myself to be bisexual. At first, I thought I was only going through a phase. I masturbated while looking at pictures from magazines and catalogs and pretended these people were my lovers. I figured I would grow out of this, but then I fell in love with a woman I worked with. Her name was Audrey, and she was exquisite. I fantasized about her a lot until she moved away and got married.

I am extremely turned on by men kissing and having sex. I'm not sure how this came about, but nothing gets me wetter. I saw an old gay porno film at a friend's house and came several times during the movie (without even touching myself—a first!). I was very aroused by the star, Joey Stefano, who died a long time ago of an overdose but had a gorgeous face and body and intense eyes and appears to love getting fucked by a man, even though there were rumors he was straight.

At the time, I was hopelessly in love with a man who lived in my apartment complex named Alan. No matter how hard I tried to get him to go out with me, he gently rebuffed my advances. My best friend told me she thought he was gay, and a lot of other people agreed. I didn't want to take him out of my fantasies completely, so I changed them to accommodate his homosexuality and still get me off!

In the fantasy, I go to Alan's for his twenty-fifth birthday party. After the presents have been opened and the last guests have gone, he asks me to stay for coffee. He breaks down in tears, and with great concern, I ask what's wrong. He tells me that he's gay and has never had a man, and it's depressing him. He doesn't want to go to bars, so I tell him not to worry—I have someone perfect in mind. I call Joey Stefano and ask him to come over.

Soon, Joey arrives, wearing a white T-shirt, black jeans, and motorcycle boots. The attraction between Joey and Alan is immediately obvious. I stand up and say, "Well, I'd better go." Joey asks me to stay and watch the fun. Now how could I refuse an offer like that?

We all go into the bedroom, and I sit on a chair while Joey and Alan fall onto the bed, French-kissing passionately. Joey unbuttons Alan's jeans and pulls at his huge, hard, throbbing cock. He sucks it and licks his balls *until Alan cums, spraying semen all over his chest. Then, Alan returns the favor, deep-throating Joey. After that, Joey and Alan take turns fucking each other in the ass, and they collapse into each other's arms.*

I get up to go, but they hear me and ask me to stay. I walk over to the bed, and they tell me to strip. I lean back against Alan, and Joey drops to his knees at the foot of the bed. "Here's to the start of a beautiful friendship!" he says and starts flicking my clit with his talented tongue. As I pump my hips, grinding my cunt against Joey's face, Alan caresses my breasts and nuzzles my hair and neck. I cum, screaming their names.

JEALOUSY

In reality, I'd suggest not diminishing the possibility of being left out in a trio. Nothing puts a soggier damper on a hot sex scene than that old "Why are they having such a good time and not including me?" We've pictured the threesome in our mind, just so, where we "pull the strings." "They" move and do exactly what we wish, precisely as we see and feel the scene, written, directed, and starred in by us. Here is the beauty of fantasy, our very own home movie where we are the master/mistress of all that happens in this little scenario in our head.

But what if they aren't acting in reality like they do in our fantasy? "Hey, you two, remember me, the star of this picture? Why am I on the cutting room floor?" Have you seen your beloved going down on another person? Maybe you have in fantasy where you control everything. So, forget about reality. If your imagination goes to threesomes and you are pleasured by the site of two, or desire to be pleasured by two, follow the leads of people in this chapter—and enjoy!

Alas, in reality, erotic trios can't help but turn into various one-on-ones. Think of when you were young and three of you played together. It wasn't unusual for us girls to leave out one. It didn't begin that way, but the temptation was there, a seed often planted by parents who favored one child over another, though they would deny it.

Even if the three of us talk it through so that everyone knows the script, their part, who can foresee what may happen when each is on his or her own erotic trip? Once the blood starts heating up, two of the three can start seeing one another with new eyes, new fingers and body parts, and before you know it, the trio has turned into a duet, leaving the third party a voyeur of sorts.

Sometimes, the voyeur doesn't get a big bang out of it. Those of us who'd rather not get involved in a threesome very often have memories of being left out of the childhood "romance"; others simply know too well the grim pang of jealousy. Sometimes, it's not another child that is favored but the intense, tight relationship between the parents that doesn't leave room for the child. To be a voyeur of your parents' love affair can leave its mark. The grim pang of jealousy when one is young, does it ever really go away? Even later on, when a mate is faithful, suspicion is still there. A fantasy of either watching or being part of a trio would be hell.

Being the third wheel of my mother and sister had its toll. For those of us who never want to be left out again, we choreograph in fantasy our little party of three so that we get everything we desire. Sometimes, the third party watches, which can be fun for either the performer or the voyeur. Sometimes, all hell breaks loose. Our beloved gets jealous, decks the other guy, and carries us off in triumph up to a blessed orgasm.

We are so defined sexually—our feelings about our body, what we can and can't let ourselves do sexually—all from a time we often don't remember. But these secret memories are the keys to what brings us to the erotic edge, until we are let go like a wild kite on a string no longer attached to this Earth.

But do not denigrate jealousy. It is part of our survival instinct. In an appropriate jealous situation, you want to feel the green-eyed monster, want to open your eyes if you are actually in the position of losing your beloved. However, overreacting to jealousy may be the surest way of pushing that lover away, just as the survival instinct "fear" sometimes ends up killing you. A sexual get-together of three people will not lead to the loss of one person's beloved…usually.

So, let us honor this meaningful emotion and try to understand its impact on us. Remember, a threesome fantasy is a scene in our heads alone, which need never see the light of day unless we are 100% certain we can handle it.

Emma

I am twenty-six years old, married with one child, and I am an exhibitionist. I love to show off my body, but at times, I am shy, too. I love to go around without a bra and panties; if I can get away with it, I sometimes go to work without these items. I have a clean-shaven pussy. My husband doesn't like hairy ones.

My husband calls me his little nymphomaniac. My favorite fantasy is having two men at the same time. I told my husband of this fantasy, and he agreed to let me live it out to see what it would be like. I loved it at first, but then it kind of threw me that my husband and the male friend who joined us enjoyed watching each other so much. I felt like waving my hands, saying, "Hey, guys, I'm over here." I'm not saying I won't ever do another threesome. I just won't do it with my husband.

SHARING ONE MAN
"A Hard Man Is Good to Find"

We women have our problems to contend with, but no one expects our clitoris to stand at erection. Men have more at stake imagining themselves in a threesome with a woman and another man. For a woman who can handle jealousy, sharing her man can be a sensational piece of pie. She's often shared a bed with another female, first mother, then sleepovers with other young girls, and now this lovely woman in bed with her and her man.

How interesting to imagine in fantasy or to actually live out a scene wherein she watches her husband with her friend, seeing herself in the other woman's place to the extent that she can almost feel what the other woman is feeling, having been there. And how is he, her man, feeling with this new woman? Without the nasty "grrrr" of jealousy, perhaps she's able to assist her man in pleasing this lovely woman. And if that works out, perhaps switch places with the woman without skipping a beat or switch to a duo wherein the other woman now watches her and her husband do the erotic dance they do so well. Though now, with eyes upon them, they perform as never before, feeling the intensity of the other woman's gaze, the sheer exhibitionism of it all!

For the men and women in this chapter, a threesome fantasy is a ticket to the World Series. In our erotic imaginations, we move the other two players around at will, picturing our best friend bringing our husband to a climax, or maybe the friend bringing us to climax while he watches and masturbates, or maybe—?

Sasha

We know men often like the scene of their woman aroused by either another woman or a man. "Let me take you in. Let me look! Let me *see!*" Watching one's mate can be a rich turn-on. Now more and more women are joining the club. Sasha dreams of including another woman with her and her fiancé, with her dream scene being the sight of her lover filling every orifice of another woman.

My fantasy is that I'd love to have a girl with my fiancé Max and me, where we all have sex. I want to see Max lick her cunt, fuck her in her ass, and make her cum. I want to go down on her and taste her pussy, feel her juices on my tongue and all over my face, making me sticky. I want her to lick my pussy so I can know what another woman *feels and tastes like. Max knew about my fantasy, and we talked about it during sex. It drove us crazy with wanting. The only problem was, we didn't know where to find another willing woman. We were both hesitant to go online, but a few months ago, our desire finally got the best of us. We've been sharing a beautiful woman ever since. Thank you, Internet!*

Perhaps the fact that Sasha had been sexually active with both men and women from an early age assuages some of the insecurity others might feel in her dream scene.

WOMEN ON TOP

The old line that men "needed" sex in a way that we women did not is quickly becoming an old wives' tale or, perhaps more appropriately, an "old husbands'" tale. Women today are going places we didn't used to even (literally) fantasize about. After depriving ourselves of our full sexuality for so long, our entrance into the workplace has everything to do with our sexual acceptance of who we are and what we want. I might add that a threesome is relatively new for women. Amazing what real independence can do for the imagination.

horny lena — 21

Hullo boys I am a 21 year old bisexual prison officer. I am looking for lads to go out with, have a few drinks and a laugh. I am single, like both sexes, but prefer men. I love to travel, eat out, not into cinema. I prefer pubs & clubs. My fantasy is to have a threesome with another guy and girl but I am not sure if I would go through with it.

3SOME WW + 1 M — 35 (woman+woman+male)

Let loose, come party tonight with me and my friend who is a guy. 420 (marijuana) and drinks, and whatever else.

both black, me, bbw (big beautiful woman) female, he very slim, dark, handsome and great in bed.

lets have fun tonight. SAFE PLAY ONLY ALWAYS

i can host i live alone, nice apartment.

hit me if you are interested.

oh and yes I'm bi, so you should be too.

2 BBw's Seeking A 3rd BBw Playmate Tonight (Our Place)

Playful and sexually adventurous, uninhibited professional femme lesbian BBw's (Big Beautiful Woman) looking for another experienced serious BBw to join us in a 3some TONIGHT, the pleasure will be very satisfying.

Knowing that your sexually safe with excellent hygiene allows us to enjoy our playtime/great sex. We are both d&d (drug & disease) free and clean so approach us correctly ladies.

Not here to play email tag or picture games with you all evening we value our time and we're serious about meeting TONIGHT.

Be ready to voice verify…exchange pictures… and meet/travel.

LADIES ONLY

Any college girls want to get together? — 22

I'm moving away soon so want to have fun before I do. Always wanted to a try 3some with 2 other women. NO MEN please. If any girls interested, I can arrange it and host.

Only clean, drug free, sweet. Any race ok.

Write about yourself and send picture if you can. Thanks.

THE GAY MAN'S *LACK OF* GUIDE TO PLEASURE

From online personal ads, I find frightening the amount of dangerous unprotected sex going on amongst young gay men. The endless ads demanding "BB" or "Raw" (bareback/no condom) make me want to grab them by the ears and shake some sense into them. Though the majority of gay men may act responsibly, dangerous sex is much more rampant in the gay population than heterosexual or lesbian. I'm not surprised. We women have been taught to say "No!" How many gay men are raised to value their homosexuality? Still today, so many parents put out signals to dissuade their child from anything but a heterosexual life. Without the love, support, and guidance, where do we learn to appreciate and care for who we are? How can we act appropriately if we have never been encouraged to be comfortable with our sexuality, a most essential part of our being?

looking for threesome – double fuck – 28

i wanna get on my knees and have two guys fuck me at the same time planting their seed… getting off on the idea of double

i am white, 6´ tall, 160lbs, 30˝ waist, 28yo, br hr hz eyes, hiv neg/std free

like to get head, give head, rim and fuck, get fucked…nice ass and legs, can host…send stats AND a pic and be around my age and hot… vers masc…at home after a fun night, horny as hell, be musc and straight-acting, ready for sex into white and black musc toned, masc guys…

really into tight ass and big arms…wrestlers and jocks a plus!

looking for a daddy bear to be a host tonight – 22

My friend i need a hairy raw top guy to host us tonight. If you can host a threesome, email me now with pic and stats and location. Must be a nice guy, very discreet, drug and disease free.

I need a 3some – 28

Im a good looking Puerto Rican top (meaning "dominant") looking for a 3some. Im looking for 2 hot older white guys who can host. Guys can be a couple, friends, fuck buddies what ever. Im not looking to steal anyones love, partner, fuck buddy. im just looking to help another top fuck a nice raw bttm. I prefer older couple but older man younger bttm or younger top and older bttm will work. Married guy here discreet, your pic gets mine. Im D&D free. Not talking about body pics here. Im looking for face pic trades. not into endless emails please.

THE GAY/LESBIAN WITHIN

A threesome sounds like so much fun. The word itself promises a good time, the more the merrier. Who doesn't like a party—especially when ice cream and balloons are replaced with hot forbidden sex? We go into it ready to double the pleasure, double the fun.

But as I discovered from my own first experience, sometimes

there is another reason for creating the party of three, one that the hosts and guests are often reluctant to admit, even to themselves. Consider the bisexual, or latent homosexual, who is drawn to a same-sex union but hasn't yet consummated it. Given shyness, fear, anxiety, uncertainty as to whether he or she can handle it, it's not uncommon for men and women to live out a same-sex experience through their partner/spouses. A suppressed homosexual wish? Or could we settle for ardent erotic curiosity?

THE BUDDY SYSTEM
Buddies! Pals! Bisexuals?

Earl

Earl, a married man in his mid-thirties, is deeply aroused by videos of his wife doing everything with four men. He fantasizes his wife being fucked to the breaking point by an enormous black man. In another email, he also fantasizes about a sixteen-year-old girl in a threesome with two men who fill every orifice, "filling (the girl) completely with their cum." In actuality, he lost his virginity to his mother's best friend. Is he gay? Does he long to be in his wife's position, every orifice filled? Clearly, a three-way with his wife and another man excites him. But is the female presence necessary to his sexual arousal, or there to cover his bisexuality? Does even he know?

I knew, and approved, of my wife's "promiscuity" before our marriage. She told me everything, though not in detail. However, two years into it, I stumbled on some old videotapes, genuine homemade porno with my wife the star! I felt cheated. Not because she hadn't told me but because she'd never done those things with me. I have to admit watching those tapes got me hot as hell. Watching my wife having four guys, seeing them in her ass and pussy at the same time, hearing her cries of pleasure as they showered her with their semen, brought on many a fine load.

I sometimes now fantasize watching my wife with a huge black man. He's so big, my wife's fingers can't encircle his thickness. I tell her that I want to watch her suck his cock. I watch as the man grabs a handful of my wife's hair, holds her head, and fucks her face. Spit dribbles from her wide-stretched lips. She can't swallow fast enough. By the time he has all of his meat inside her pussy, she's biting her lip in pain, unable to concentrate on kissing me, but she keeps right on fucking him back. Her eyes meet mine, pleading for intervention. As they glaze over, I know she's cumming. He fucks her to the limits of her endurance as he drives his cock deep and dumps his load inside her.

Meosha

A twenty-seven-year-old black mother of two, Meosha is engaged to be married. She did not get a chance to go to college but thinks she may do that once her kids are a little older.

My sex drive has always been unbelievable. I can remember being five and playing house with my cousins. We were too young to take off our clothes, so we just lay on top of each other and ground our little bodies together. But my mom found us and told us we were nasty and punished us. Funny thing is, I always used to see my parents kissing and touching each other's body parts. My sister and brother used to giggle every time we heard the springs in my parents' bed making noise.

My favorite fantasy starts like this. One hot July day, I get upset with my boyfriend, and I jump in my car to leave, with no destination in mind. I end up at an adult movie theater, dressed scantily for the summer, and two women sit down on either side of me—one a blonde, the other a brunette.

The movie is about two roommates, talking about their boyfriends, when one grabs the other's breast and squeezes the nipple. Her friend smiles and says she has always wanted to do the same to her. At this moment, myself and the ladies on each side of me sigh with excitement. The next thing I know, the blonde next to me asks if I would get upset if she sucked my pussy. "Now?" I say. "Yes," she says. Slowly, she kneels down between my legs and slides her head between my thighs and starts to kiss my swollen clit ever so softly. At the same time, the brunette leans over and asks if she can stroke my breast. Keeping my eyes on the screen, watching the women bring each other to climax, I too reach an earth-shattering orgasm. We end up at a sauna, where we have a hot threesome.

Jacques

A twenty-four-year-old man, educated at a prestigious college, with a major in philosophy, Jacques has been with his partner, Catherine, for over six years. He says he is now paying off his college loans working as a temp. "It's so Generation X, you could puke," he comments.

I tell you, Catherine is everything a man could hope for sexually. I've never made a demand that she has not accommodated to sooner or later. Our lovemaking is varied and interesting, with a lot of different positions. She's fulfilled just about every fantasy that I have had involving two people. My fantasies now, therefore, involve more than just the two of us. Something I would love to do for her is let her enjoy two men at once. I may never overcome my hang-ups enough to allow this fantasy to actually happen, but it will always excite me as a fantasy.

The other man in the fantasy is a friend of ours, someone whom we are both close to. The occasion is not forced; there are no heavy expectations. It just happens naturally—in a hot tub or nude sunbathing, something like that. We begin by expressing our love in a way that seems natural in front of him. He, in fact, encourages this. When we look over at him, he has a hard-on. This gives us all the permission we need. I take the plunge, laying her on her back, spreading her legs wide, and bury my face in her pussy. I am going wild, trying to kiss, lick, and touch every soft, velvety inch of her vulva. Her clit is throbbing, and she is bucking her hips. Then, she swings around so we are in a 69 position, and she immediately takes my cock in her mouth as far as it will go, while she pulls down on my ass.

I come up for air and look at our friend, who is jerking off. For me, it is the first cock I have seen raging for action. We both like to watch. After a while, she gets on her knees, and I slide my iron-hard rod into her dripping wet cunt from behind so that we're both facing him. He is looking at us like he wishes he weren't alone. He starts to talk to us, telling us what good fuckers we are, telling me to screw her and her to fuck the jism out of me.

But I'm not ready for that. I want this to last, so I ease up a little and ask her if she likes the looks of Bernie's penis. "Yes, yes," she says, so I ask her if she wants to touch it. When Bernie indicates he is not opposed, she crawls over to where he is lying and takes his dick in her hands, feeling the shape of the corona and head. Finally, when he can't stand it any longer, she takes the thing in her mouth. The sight of her head bobbing up and down has me almost cumming right there. Her ass is straight up in the air, and I return to fucking her doggie style.

Finally, I tell her to get on top of him. She crawls up and lowers herself onto his cock. The clear view of her fucking another guy with gusto is mind-blowing. I have to be a part of this, so I push my cock gently into her ass, and we're all three fucking away like there's no tomorrow. We're all one big writhing mass of carnal flesh.

Victor

I'm a lapsed Catholic, now into Eastern religions, and pretty happily married. I know my wife is turned on by men. She fantasizes about her boss and some very sexy black men she's met. I think it's healthy and very important to know her sexual nature, and frankly, it's also a turn-on for me to know that my wife is an independent, highly evolved, sexual human being.

I'm basically heterosexual. However, I've had hot sex with gay and bisexual men in the past. Alone and in groups. Though I find women very, very sexually attractive, fucking or sucking another man is a special turn-on for me. I fantasize about having an iron-hard man stand above me, in a bathtub, and urinate on me while I masturbate.

Now on to my favorite fantasy. This part is true: My bisexual friend Darcy—my best man at our wedding and a member of a Sufi spiritual community—is tall, well-built, and possesses a large cock. He enjoys giving full body massages to both sexes. My fantasy is that Darcy visits our house on a summer weekend. After a shared lunch with copious amounts of wine, we step out onto our secluded patio. We all strip off our clothing. Darcy sets up his massage table next to the hot tub. Alexis, my wife, asks for him to massage her first. I agree and step into the hot tub to relax and look across our lawn to the pine-covered Rocky Mountains, just four miles away.

On her stomach, Alexis is clearly in ecstasy. She is aroused and squirms gently under Darcy's masculine touch. After about five minutes, he asks her if she would feel comfortable with him manually stimulating her clit. She nods yes. He slips a hand under her to grab her mound of hair, then jiggles her clit to a point when she responds with the aroused sigh of a sex slave under her master's firm hand. Then, he politely asks her if he may eat her pussy from behind. She turns her head and looks at me for unquestioning approval. What can I say? I agree and support her adventure in paradise.

He starts lapping her soaked cunt, and she approaches a climax. Darcy slides his tongue up from her vagina and begins to lick her perineum. Then, he parts both her ass cheeks and begins tongue-fucking her anus. Of course, my cock is now rock-hard. I masturbate myself vigorously.

In an instant, Alexis cums in spasms. "I've never, never felt this kind of intensity before. It was an amazingly different kind of fuck," she mutters breathlessly. She says I must experience Darcy's magic fingers. "You'll love it, and you know it."

Darcy oils me and lathers the lavender oil around my penis and testicles and begins to masturbate me slowly. While he does this, Alexis steps behind him and grabs some oil. I see her begin to masturbate Darcy with her right hand. Darcy grabs my erect cock and spreads apart the tiny, fleshy lips at the opening of my urethra. He begins darting the tip of his tongue in and out of my now swollen pisshole. A fountain of milky cum arcs into the air and onto Darcy's chin, which hovers just above my glans. He jerks up, surprised at the shot, and laughs with delight.

Alexis is still masturbating him. My friend shoots his load on my pubic hair and navel. I feel a bond of our spent seed.

Lily

I'm twenty-one, a dental assistant, heterosexual, but I really enjoy being what people think of as the life of the party. I've had numerous one-night stands. Something that really turns me on is that the men always make the first move. I don't like being dominant.

My fantasy doesn't actually involve me. It's basically one hell of an orgy. I will describe the acts only briefly, as I am on the train at the moment and can't exactly go and walk off in a corner somewhere.

It starts with two lesbians who have had a long-standing relationship. They haven't seen each other for a while, so as soon as they do, they are damp with excitement. They start kissing and fingering each other. (I'm not a lesbian, but thinking about lesbian sex turns me on.) Let's call them Iris and Yvette. They are rubbing their cunts madly together and bringing each other to orgasm when Yvette's cousin, Stuart, and his wife Blanche knock at the door. They have come around for a drink. After a few beers, Blanche admits she would like to try sex with a woman. They begin to play strip poker and things get a little hot. Yvette rips Blanche's g-string off, licks her nipples until they are hard and erect. She then licks her clitoris until she cums all over her face. Iris and Stuart watch this and get very horny. They have sex until they cum everywhere.

The three women then have sex together using a vibrator on each other. Iris and Yvette then get into a 69, while Blanche uses the vibrator on herself. They all have wonderful orgasms. Stuart gets really hard while he is watching all this and wants to get in on the action. He goes over to Yvette and shoves his cock into her mouth. She gives him a blow job, while the women lick her streaming cunt.

Wondering.....Guys Would Love 2 Women But Do Women Want 2 Men?

Hi ladies.

For as long as time, I would bet 95% (or more) of the guys on this planet would kill to have 2 women at a time and experience a MFF (male-female-female) threesome.

So.......is the opposite true? Do women secretly fantasize about having 2 men at their disposal? Does the idea of a str8 guy with another str8 guy and you sound erotic?

This WM 39, is well.....very curious!

Double Your Pleasure?

Ok, my buddy and I were in Atlantic City a few months back and somehow ended up in a 3some with a hot chick. At first I didn't want to do it but long story short is we did, and I have to admit it was a lot hotter than I thought it would be! Just everything about it was hot, taking turns on her, watching her get it from all angles brought out the voyeur/exhibitionist in both of us.

What we're looking for is another girl that would like to be taken by 2 hot guys with big equipment. Yes, we are both rather well endowed so please like it that way. Both of us are Caucasian.

Guy #1 is a 30 year old, very fit, with blue eyes and a powerful build, rugged good looks

and specialties include: banging your g-spot,
and slow licking you wherever you like it most.

Guy #2 is a 27 year old, fit body dark hair
and blue eyes, who loves taking you from behind
while you suck on a nice size dick.

Both men are gracious, always respectful of
your limits and d/d free.

Please be attractive!

For some of us, a third person "takes the edge off." I'm reminded of the old "buddy" movies where the one guy, a young Frank Sinatra, is shy and only feels safe approaching women when his more worldly pal, a smooth Gene Kelly, is along. If something goes wrong, if it doesn't work out, if the woman rejects him/them, well, it's not because he's a loser. If she doesn't want to join in, tough luck. Who needs her? I've got my buddy. There's always another dame just around the corner. I can have just as much fun with my pal.

The nice thing about a three-way is that you can enjoy living out the fantasy without making any extreme decision as to your "true" sexual identity. But then, why does it have to be either/or, straight or gay? Women haven't been hard-pressed to label themselves "lesbian" because they've had sex with a woman. Shall we let men off the hook, drop the label, and just let them "be"?

If people let go of their fear of comparison, the anxiety at being rejected, they can enjoy a fantasy that gets them close to the erotic self they feel is inside them; this is what fantasy can/ should do. The obstacle, of course, is that too many of us think the thought is the deed.

Isn't "not ever knowing" worse than giving yourself over to erotic fantasy and asking yourself, "Is this, was this, something I'd really like to try?" Fantasies aren't road maps we are directed to follow; they simply tell us that these images and plots are what bring us to orgasm. It's a rocky road sometimes because there are ancient obstacles along the way, laid there largely by parental control when we were young and malleable.

Imagine your fantasies as x-rays of your libido. Once upon a time, it was strong, healthy, full of potential. Along the way, various people messed with it. Not everyone's libido is the same, but they all want to be sexually thriving. That's what your vivid imagery is telling you, not always that you really want to do these things but that you want to feel erotically alive. The beauty of fantasy is that you can be with anyone. Mother will never know.

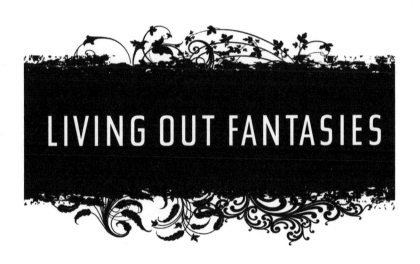

LIVING OUT FANTASIES

LIVING OUT FANTASIES

Sometimes, the urge to live out a fantasy is so intense, it's unbearable. Nothing can take us from this Earth, lift us to another realm, like that sexual longing we crave. It comes from the deepest recesses of our being. Perhaps this is why, along with the computer advertising swift speed to realizing our erotic dreams, we're led to situations in contrast to the person we are, a person of sense and reason.

There is something foreboding about approaching someone or calling on the phone and either getting voice mail, being put on hold, or simply being rejected flat out. With the Internet, you can approach dozens of prospects in no time. If they don't respond, send a rejection, block you, it's not you. It's a profile/picture, hardly the beautiful soul you emanate in person. And for all you know, they've rejected you because they aren't the hot blonde chick they've advertised, they're Reese, our sixty-five-year-old slender gay man, who is sexually seducing handsome men online around the world.

The lowering of limits on what is sexually doable and living with less prudery and Puritanism have helped us become an age of instant gratification. Even if you can't afford what you desire, the message is out there that others are into it, having it, loving it, adding envy to our consumer sex-crazed world. Little good can be said of envy other than the force it has to drive us.

As I've said, be careful when conjuring a fantasy into reality. It's delicate magic that can leave wondrous to devastating results. But in no way am I discouraging you, only advising to check carefully before diving in head first. Make sure it's hot enough for you to be comfortable when totally immersed. For some, it is everything they've dreamed and more.

THE DREAM COMES TRUE

Every now and then, I hear from someone who touches my own erotic nerve. Such was the case with Vanessa. Years ago, she'd met a man she was particularly attracted to. He said he'd call. Time passed, and he didn't. The fantasies began, erotic trips of what might have been. Haven't we all been there?

Vanessa

I am a fifty-seven-year-old, twice-divorced single mother of two children and grandmother of six. I have enjoyed a very wonderful sex life and the fulfillment of many fantasies in the past thirty-plus years. I have been living alone now for the past two years, and I had decided that my sex life, as I had known it in the past, was probably over. About a month ago, I bumped into an old male friend. I used to fantasize about him when I was with my lover at the time. I knew I would never be able to really have that sexual experience with him, but he was in many of my fantasies over the years. When I met him again, he asked me if I was still in a relationship, and I said no.

Then, one day, I went into my office, and there was a voice message on the phone from him. We started emailing back and forth, and he wrote that he thought these emails were going to get sexual. We started fantasizing, and I started telling him things about parts of my life that I knew would turn him on. A few days later, he left me an erotic voice mail. He told me exactly how he was going to lick me and suck me. It was then that he asked me if I trimmed down there or, better yet, did I shave? I played that voice mail over and over when I was alone with my vibrator just to cum to his voice.

We continued to email, and I finally asked him, "Do you think we will ever really get together?" His answer was, "Of course. Why do you think we're doing all this?" Then, on Monday morning, I went into work, and there was an email from him: "WHAT ARE YOU DOING TONIGHT?"

When he called me on the phone just before he got to my house, he asked me one question: "Are you ready for me?" Oh, I was ready for him. He came into my house and gave me a sweet kiss hello. We shared a joint that he had brought over, and he leaned over to me and asked me if I was nervous. I said yes and then he said the most extraordinary thing: "I am too."

I think that was all we needed. He was a wonderful lover. Oh, reality does beat fantasy at times. He had a beautiful cock, and I loved sucking on it. When it became flaccid, I took it in my mouth and sucked on it until it grew hard and so delicious. Then, he put it in my cunt and fucked me until I was soaking wet with need and want. Then, he turned me over and entered me from behind. That was enough to just make me burst wide open. He was so deep inside of me and thrusting forward even more deeply that it was the most delicious feeling. Afterward, I couldn't believe that I had actually had this wonderful intimate sexual experience with the man I had always enjoyed in my fantasies. Not only is he a great lover, but he's also an interesting, exciting man to talk to.

My children and grandchildren probably think the most stimulating thing we do is watch **Wheel of Fortune.** *But maybe being forbidden makes it all the more exciting. I've had a wonderful time with him, and the only question I'm left with, and I wonder if it's a female thing, is will he continue to see me? Boy, I hope so.*

Sydney

I'm a twenty-five-year-old, well-educated professional working with and for the positive behavior in schools initiative. I came out to the world and my family two years ago, and I'm extremely happily married to my wonderful partner, Sylvia.

When I was about seven years old, my cousin showed me how to masturbate my clitoris and how to use candles inside to feel good. We "played" every time we were together. We knew that if our parents found out they might make us stop, so we were careful not to let them in on our secret. We didn't see that there was anything dirty or bad with what we were doing because neither of us had been taught any type of hate or bad feelings about sex at that age. I might add at this point that my mother is and was an out-lesbian. It made no difference to my upbringing, which was fairly average considering my mother.

One day, when I was about eleven, I was alone in the house. I was reading the titles of books on the shelf by my mother's bed, and I saw your book. My Secret Garden. *I recognized the title as a children's book, so I picked it up and read the back cover. I was hooked. I remember that day very well indeed. I lay on my momma's bed, reading your book, touching myself, and without realizing, I came extremely close to orgasm. I put the book down by my side and "finished myself off" for the first time. I realized that people out there did and thought much more extreme things than this eleven-year-old girl. I also got the sense that I could explore—and it wasn't wrong.*

My mother later said that she had known exactly what I had been doing but that she respected my right to explore by myself.

I didn't have penetrative sex until later in life—at about eighteen—because I didn't need to. I managed very well on my own, thank you very much. When I did have sex with a man for the first time, it did nothing for me. To be honest, it was a bit boring. I started to fantasize more and more about women and in comes another of your books, Women on Top. *This time, it was brought as a present by my boyfriend of the time. I read it, and my fantasies about women were abated.*

After some years exploring myself and three or four men, I had a relationship with a woman. It was everything I had dreamed of and more (which is saying something). I continued relationships with women in private for quite some time. I tried out the BDSM scene and found that interesting for a while. Then I met Sylvia. I am now very happy living with her in a stable relationship. I know I have tried everything I ever wanted to where sex is concerned. I still fantasize and masturbate.

I now have a healthy alternative lifestyle over which I have no remorse or guilt. I am content that I have explored myself and all possibilities and now I am more than ready to commit myself to sex with just one woman. I doubt I will ever wonder if the grass is greener elsewhere because I know the difference between reality and fantasy. I also understand that it is possible to go where I want in my head without fear of it being wrong or abnormal. And that I can act out some of my fantasies within my relationship just for the fun of it.

I love the fact that although I am the more feminine one in our relationship, I can still pick Sylvia up and carry her to our bedroom. If I want, I am free to "play" the more dominant role, act the innocent little girl, or be the sex kitten wearing sexy clothes. I can play the slave girl and wash, dry, and dress Sylvia. I am also very comfortable "playing" whatever role Sylvia wants. I can breast-watch and still be faithful to her—we often do it together. The point is that I am free, and if I was so inclined, I wouldn't feel any shame in thinking about men, animals, household objects, my brother, or aliens.

Stefan

I'm now fifty-one and seldom masturbate, though I did frequently as a boy. I still have a lot of varied fantasies, though, which I use mainly while making love to my wife. I occasionally make love to other women, some girlfriends, and some prostitutes and make much slighter use of fantasies on these occasions.

Most of my fantasies are based upon a woman I know, whom I find attractive, but I know wouldn't normally have sex with me. It starts where I have to sacrifice something, like money or my marriage, in order to get her to sleep with me. She can get me to do anything. Very soon, she wants other lovers. I have to set it up, but I'm driven crazy with jealousy and want her even more.

I watch her get involved in threesomes with other couples that I know. And sometimes I have to buy her a dog for her to have sex with.

This suggests that I like to be humiliated, and indeed, some element of humiliation seems necessary to bring me to orgasm. As I'm getting older and never had a partner who tried to humiliate me during sex, I realized it may never happen. So, I finally confessed to my wife, and to my surprise, she agreed to it. She said she'd always felt there was something missing. She wouldn't let me watch her in a threesome, but she was more than happy to humiliate me. I was pretty amazed what a pro she was at it. Whatever anger and disgust she had felt toward me during all the years we've been together came pouring out. It was an incredible turn-on. However, we haven't done it again yet. We might just leave it as a special one-time thing or maybe a special once-a-year thing for my birthday. Who knows? But I'm definitely up for it.

Jill

I have always had sexual fantasies. As far as I know, I've been having them since I was five years old. I'm now twenty-four but can remember sneaking upstairs to look at a photo album that my parents had hidden. It had pictures of them in all sorts of sexual positions, and I remember getting certain feelings from looking at it.

I now live out every fantasy that I can. My favorite is when my boyfriend throws me on the bed and undresses me. Then, he turns me over so that my bottom faces up. He ties my hands and puts handcuffs on my wrists. Then, he starts to spank me while smoking his pipe. (Pipe smoke turns me on.) Then, he starts to lick me from behind. That is the best eating out that I have ever felt. He grabs my ass and pulls it up close to his cock and shoves it in me as hard as he can till I cum.

We take a shower, and he shoves it in me again. Finally, I tell him I have to go pee, and he lets me but plays with my clit as I do so. That is the best orgasm ever. After I'm done, I stand, and he licks my pussy, telling me how good I taste and how hot and wet I was.

Dru

I come from a fanatically religious upbringing. My father tried to control my life even after I was married. I'm divorced now and have three children. My mother, although a successful businesswoman, never discussed sex with my sister or me. In fact, I don't think I ever heard her utter the word.

My first sexual experience at twenty got me pregnant. The boy disappeared, and, of course, I married an obsessive, controlling, abusive ass just like my father. That lasted, incredibly, thirteen years. The day after my third daughter was born, I had a hysterectomy. And the day she started kindergarten, I left. It was hard, but I raised them alone.

After a pretty tough time, including operations and ulcers, I met the man I thought didn't exist. We now live on a farm. Raise our own vegetables, goats, chickens, and rabbits. I said all that to lead up to the best part. Before I met Ronnie, he had had a lot of women. They even used to send their friends to him, two or three at a time. So, even though he was gentle, the sex overwhelmed me. But for the first time, I became orgasmic.

It took five years into the marriage before I told Ronnie that I had fantasies about a threesome with another woman. He got excited and went out and found one.

I knew I'd enjoy seeing him "do" another girl, but I had no idea what it would do to me. I was on the bottom, she was licking me, and he was behind her by then. The harder he pumped her, the harder she licked me. We were all three carrying on like animals. I reached up and grabbed his beautiful buttocks and pulled him deeper into her. My fantasies were good, but reality tops everything I ever imagined.

Real scenes that might have disgusted us twenty years ago are fodder for tonight's erotic fantasy. Take that stranger across from us on the bus. He caught us staring unknowingly at the enormous bulge in his trousers. When had our eyes gone there? Chagrined, we get off the bus before our accustomed stop, quickly turn and see him staring at us from the window, his tongue lasciviously licking his lips, then showing us how his tongue will lick our clitoris. We quickly turn away in disgust.

But not so disgusted that we don't put him and that tongue into our fantasy at night as we lie beside our sleeping mate. A mate so very dear but known far too well for the kind of forbidden sex we desire, the kind of dirty sex the vile stranger would force upon us.

As I, and more than one person in this book, have admitted, there can be a downside to living out a fantasy. In fantasy, we control everyone and everything like Olympian gods. Once we've invited others to play out this theme that never fails to give us orgasmic pleasure, these real-life people don't always respond as we would have them.

Being made to feel inferior, smaller, unworthy can be a sexual turn-on for some, if executed properly. But even most masochists desire the attention drawn on them. They are the ones worthy of being punished, abused, humiliated.

If I pay someone to force me to snivel at their feet, and instead, I'm forced to sit in a corner watching someone else take the abuse, I'll want my money back. For many, nothing makes a penis droop or a vagina dry and wither like jealousy. So, as I advised with threesomes, think twice about living out your fantasy.

KILLING THE DREAM

It is always a toss-up, this business of trying in real life what excites us in our imagination. While it is thrilling in fantasy to fuck another person while our married mate watches, we can't "stage manage" reality as we do our fantasy. We can't force our partner's eyes to stay focused on us instead of this new woman or man folded into this supposed dream come true.

For some, the reason not to tell our mate the fantasy that most excites us isn't just a question of our beloved's response but the added risk that once aired, the fantasy might be less exciting the next time that we call upon it. Secrecy is often the spice that keeps the oldest and dearest fantasies fresh as the day they were born. Living out a fantasy, even telling it, can lessen the erotic impact forever.

The following fantasies in this chapter show some of the many reasons fantasies are sometimes best left to the imagination. For Brad, it's the remorse he felt and the lowering of his own self-esteem.

Brad

I'm a single, college-educated professional, twenty-five years old, an only child, and reared in the suburbs by parents who never talked about sex. I masturbate regularly, usually once a day if given the chance. The most I've cum with a woman is three times in one session. I would like, though, to save my cum for a least a week and then see how many times I could perform.

Women intrigue me, attract me. I believe I could gaze for hours upon nicely shaped women, observing their gentle gestures, the drape of a blouse over a breast, the cinch of blue jeans over a hip, the fall of luxurious dark hair, strands clinging against ears and neck.

My heart goes out to women. They think about relationships a lot. Look at women's magazines. I have some sexist attitudes. I believe women should stay home with young children, if they can, and not have children out of wedlock. Does this sound naïve or ancient?

I'd like to go out with a woman who is wearing no underwear. In the shadows, I slip a hand over her buttocks, under a short skirt, a finger up her twat—wet and ready. She's walking around in public with her nipples protruding, aroused. We're driving somewhere and so horny we have to pull off the highway and go fuck in the long grass.

I'd like to tie up a woman and make her so hot she's begging, absolutely begging, for my cock—for anything—a massive dildo up her cunt and asshole.

I'm on the quiet side, but I fantasize about loud fucking, moaning, and groaning, calling out obscenities. Homosexuality does not appeal to me, although I've thought about sucking another man's cock and swallowing, a mildly stimulating fantasy. Men in general repel me sexually, though. But women are so luscious I can hardly walk by a good-looking one without a fleeting imagining of my hand behind her buttocks—bada boom!

On another musing of male power, I've had the feeling that women want to capture this power for themselves, to capture me for their own protection, for their needs of affection and human contact. This is nature, to be able to capture something, someone more powerful than yourself, someone who is physically stronger. In that way, women exert a stronger power, a quiet, almost supreme power. After all, I believe that women are calling the shots when it comes to marriage, mating, the important stuff of continuing the race. And I like to think they're all still okay with men running the rest of it, building their buildings, setting up political structures, and pulling them down again.

On a last note, I have to admit that I lived out one of my fantasies. While visiting Chicago, I saw an online ad for a sex party that I answered and then was invited. There was a woman there who was tied up (willingly) and about seven of us men jerked off on her. Some of the men were calling her things like "cum bitch," "fucking whore," etc. The reality just wasn't like the fantasy in my head. I have to admit I felt badly for her. I couldn't help but think, "What happened for her to allow herself to be treated like this?" I could tell she'd been physically and mentally abused by men, and I felt like I was adding to it, taking advantage of it. I knew I never wanted to do it again.

Cindy

Cindy, a thirty-year-old woman, married with two children, knows better than to turn one of her fantasies into reality.

I've been called every name—whore, slut, tramp. But I have never thought of it that way. Especially when the girls and guys who were saying that were doing exactly the same thing. My husband's friend— and boss—told me one night that he had a girlfriend but that when he makes love to her, he always thinks of me. This was revealed one night when he was over at our house and my husband had gone out to pick up some pot. I'd had a fantasy about him with his girlfriend and my husband in a foursome, but I fantasize about stuff like that every day. Thinking about sex is one of my favorite pastimes. However, I'm not unfaithful. I lost all that was important to me once because of that, *and I don't think I could ever do that again. The sex just wasn't worth it. I would hate to lose everything I have. I would also hate to lose my husband's trust. We just aren't ready to explore that far yet. He could get very jealous.*

Keith

Sixteen years old and a senior in high school, Keith recently returned to the United States from an all-boys school in Britain.

It was great. I had a lot of gay sex there. If there is one thing I won't run out of, it's sexual fantasies. Now that I'm back home, one of my classmates here is the focal point of my fantasies. Cameron is seventeen, and we were always out getting high or drunk, but, oh, how I wanted him! Well, it finally happened. Cam and I got a six-pack and were parked, drinking. After we were a little high, I broke the ice by asking him how much he jacks off. He says a couple of times a week. I say, "That's all?" We laugh 'cause we both know it's a lot more. I ask him if he feels like it now. He says: "I don't know. Do you?" I say, "Sure." In no time, we're out of our pants. I tell him about some of the things I did at my school in Britain, and when I'm finished, he asks kind of suspiciously if I want to get it off with him. I say: "Sure. It doesn't mean anything. It's just fun. If we're not feeling it, we can stop."

We undress all the way, and man, do I have a raging hard-on. He lays on top of me and starts licking my nipples. I can tell he's jerking off. So, I move down to service his cock with my mouth until I swallow every drop. I think that's it, so I'm ready to jerk off, but without a word, he goes down on me. He strokes me with his mouth, and in no time, I cum. I see him lick some of it off of him. He lies close to me, our bodies rubbing against each other's, and we begin French-kissing. When I get home, I jerk off a couple more times just thinking about it.

But the next day I see him, and he's acting weird, like it didn't happen, or he was too drunk to remember. Then, he keeps avoiding me. I barely see him now except in school when he doesn't have a choice. It was amazing having that fantasy actually happen with him, and I still jerk off to it. But I miss him as a friend. If I could take it back, I would. I pretty much wish it never happened. The way I feel now, it would've been better to just keep it in my head.

Benjamin

I was married for eighteen years to a very sexual girl. Karin and I enjoyed a tremendous sex life, and we had two children. But once, she was lent a porn video, which we were watching together. It was rather boring, so she went to sleep, and I stayed up. Toward the end of the film, there was a fantastic gay scene between these two hunks, and I was so turned on that I started to beat off—only to be caught in the act by Karin, who was most annoyed. Nothing more was said about it, but some months later, in London, we went into a sex shop, and she saw among the displays a strap-on dildo, complete with balls. She told me to buy it.

Back in the hotel, she told me that she wanted to fuck me, as she had seen how turned on I was watching the video. Seeing her undressed with the dildo strapped on was mind-blowing, and I readily vaselined my anus to receive her. Alas, the pain was excruciating! Though I wanted to try it, and in fact did, all the way in, I had no physical pleasure out of it and would definitely pass on it next time. However, making love to her while she still had it strapped on was fantastic.

I have a fantasy of meeting a nice, well-dressed young woman at a social function. We go to her hotel room. We start undressing, and she lays herself down on the bed, invitingly. We kiss, and I fondle her tits. She moves her hand to my own nipples and the other to my throbbing cock. The combination makes me go wild, and my hand goes for her crotch.

Then, I freeze, for there, tucked and hidden between her legs, I find a penis! My lay is a man with tits!

I go down on him/her, taking the prick in my hungry mouth, and suck it with greed. My she-male does the same to me, and as the night progresses, I fuck her ass while holding her sweet cock in my hands, bringing us both to climaxes to break all records.

For a long time, this fantasy disturbed me greatly because it gave me a complex about being gay. Now I have come to terms with myself. I understand that fantasy and reality can live side-by-side, one not disturbing the other. My fantasy of being fucked by a she-male is just that—a fantasy. I know better than to live it out. I am very much an active heterosexual man of forty-five. My eyes follow every delightful girl that passes by. Karin and I are separated now, but I look forward to meeting someone new to share a full life with.

Julissa

Julissa, a twenty-three-year-old graduate student who still lives with her parents, has fantasies about being "on top" in a sexual encounter with a man.

I come from a middle-class, fairly conservative background. I consider myself quite liberal, however, both in my political views and my personal thoughts about life.

I have many fantasies, which I use when I masturbate. They always bring me to fantastic orgasms. One is about a professor. He's not particularly attractive (funny, in my fantasies, the men are usually very plain), but in the fantasy, he's very sexy to me. I make an appointment to meet with him at his office about a paper I'm writing for his class. My appointment is in the evening, and when I arrive, the building is virtually empty. (It's great how in fantasies everything works out perfectly, isn't it?) I stand at his side while he reads my paper, and I push myself a little closer to him every minute or so. I notice that he has been on the same page for a while now, and his breathing has slowed down and gotten very heavy. Taking a chance, I put a hand on his neck and run it slowly down his back.

He closes his eyes and moans softly. Great, I know he wants me. After a minute or so of kissing my face passionately, he lifts me onto his desk and tugs at the front of my blouse. A few buttons pop off, and he groans when he sees I have no bra on. He sucks my breasts like a hungry man who hasn't eaten for days. I push his face lower and lean my torso back onto the desk. He starts to lick my cunt through the silky wet fabric of my panties. I push my cunt into his face with wild abandon, and he sucks and licks faster and faster. I look down and see he is masturbating himself while he eats me.

The sight of his hard cock in his hand makes me cum, but I still can't wait to get to his cock. I push him back into his chair and kneel at his feet. I grab his cock with both hands and start to suck it as hard as I can. He's groaning and bucking his hips to meet my mouth. I pull away from him. Then, I smile seductively and tell him I want to feel his cock inside me. I climb onto his lap and lower myself onto his ready-to-burst cock.

I move myself slowly up and down on his hard rod, milking his cock with my pussy. I start to ride him faster. We cum simultaneously, arching our backs to meet each other. I quickly dress myself, thank him for the help with the paper, and go home.

I never thought I'd have the nerve to try this in reality, but during a private evaluation in his office, he said things and gave me looks that made it clear the possibility was there. However, I just played dumb. When faced with actually having sex with him, I didn't want to. The desire wasn't there. I realized, it's only my fantasy of him that I'm attracted to, not the real person.

As we progressively remove the "forbidden" from sex, will we automatically expect the fantasy to be even more satisfying in reality? Or will some of us still give second thought to the idea that maybe all fantasies weren't meant to be aired? When a man tells his wife his fantasy of wearing women's clothes and she encourages him to put on the dress and join her for a stroll around the block, it seems endearing. But there are other sexual fantasies that aren't x-rays of what we really want to do. There's a reason they've remained only a fantasy—so far.

Nowadays, the line between fantasy and reality grows even finer. Endless email chat may eventually materialize into nothing or access to our dreams may be only a few keystrokes away. The thought becomes the deed before the consequences are weighed. Sex has become more instinct and less responsibility. We've come to think of it as disposable as any other commodity.

THE DREAM BECOMES A NIGHTMARE

Do I think the precarious state of the world today affects eros? How could it not? With the world on tilt, the possibility of obliteration is something we've learned to live with. Our fertile imaginations whip up a tailor-made fantasy to take us out of this real world and into a reflected one for that brief but oh-so-remedial orgasm.

Christine

Christine, who is twenty-two and whose brother died of AIDS, is just beginning to explore her sexuality.

I know that my boyfriend's best friend prefers women's fantasies. Is it because it is sexy to hear about the opposite sex's needs, wants, and cravings? To hear about the unknown?

As for my sexual fantasies, they run the gamut from rape fantasies to controlling men. I have an extreme fear of being raped, so my rape fantasies are strange to me. When I feel like masturbating, I review my past fantasies and select one that turns me on. If none do, I make up a brand-new one. My sexual fantasies are based more on things I've read. I get more excited by the written word than pictures (boring) or porn.

My earliest sexual fantasy was one I got from your book Men in Love, *and it still turns me on, although I've adapted it. I'm in a red Mustang convertible, driving down a lonely highway. The vibrations from the car massage my cunt, making me horny. I see a handsome young man, Will (a guy I had a serious crush on my senior year of high school). He's hitching a ride. I pick him up. We speed down the highway. He looks at me admiringly, not only because I'm pretty, tan, and my body is* hot but also because I can drive. We're going eighty miles an hour. "The curves are tricky, and unless you want to be dead," I say, "don't touch me." I'm in perfect control. I begin to masturbate with one hand as I drive with the other. It's exciting for him to watch a girl cum off because she wants to drive him crazy. I moan. My fingers dart in and out of my cunt. Suddenly, I pull the car off the road to a secluded spot. I jump out. Will scrambles after me. We fall into the long grass and make love.

I'd love this fantasy to happen, but I know it's too risky. It could end up being horrible. Still, someday, if I'm driving and see a guy like Will hitching, who knows?

Burt

I'm thirty-seven, never married, but completely heterosexual. My fantasy is admittedly very bizarre and much too dangerous to ever try out. I am walking through some open woods with three very attractive young women. We sit down and begin to play strip poker. We draw cards. Whoever gets the lowest card has to submit to anything the others wish. I lose.

They tell me to strip, and after some embarrassed hesitation, I comply. They giggle and fondle my cock, which quickly gets very hard. They order me to lie facedown on the grass, and they tie my hands behind my back. One goes away, and the other two begin to masturbate me, teasing me about how long they are going to keep me right on the edge of orgasm. The one who went away comes back with a noose and chair. They put the noose around my neck and throw the rope over a large tree limb.

I become frightened, but they tell me that they're just goofing off. They place the chair under the tree limb and tell me to stand on it. I do and then they pull down on the other end of the rope until there is absolutely no slack in it at all. They then tie the end of the rope to the trunk of the tree. The three of them walk around me, pinching my balls, caressing my ass, kissing the tip of my cock, and terrifying me by shaking the chair I am standing on.

The one who brought the noose quickly kicks the chair out from under me. All I can do is dangle there. As the realization sets in that I am slowly strangling, I panic. I begin kicking, and as I look down, one of the women is staring at me, saying, "Oh, my God, oh, my God," as she watches me jerking around in the air. But the one who tied the rope is enjoying every moment of it. She shouts, "Dance! Dance a jig for us!" My naked body bucks and jerks as my legs flail around at nothing but thin air. I struggle frantically and kick harder, but it doesn't help. My slow strangulation continues.

I hang there kicking until I am reduced to spasms and twitching, at which point they let me down. Then, the one who kicked the chair out from under me jerks me off with her hand. I shoot a tremendous quantity of cum over her hand and my own stomach.

I know where the fantasy comes from. When I was a boy, I discovered that shimmying up the slanted frame of a schoolyard swing set would rub on my cock and that it felt great. I quickly learned to fantasize that the cutest girl in my third-grade class had tied my hands and was hauling me, naked, up this slanted pipe for all the other girls to see.

Burt knows that his fantasy would not only become nightmare but could also lead to his death.

Louis

A happily married man in his early forties, Louis and his wife, Phoebe, are both teachers with advanced degrees who work in different towns and so have different groups of acquaintances. Lou had a few relationships before his marriage at twenty-four; Phoebe had more.

Our life together has been extremely happy, and we have spent many delightful hours in each other's arms. Phoebe enjoys sex greatly once we have begun foreplay, but she can go through extended periods where she has little need for it.

Phoebe takes a lot of care of her appearance and clearly enjoys male attention. She is anything but prudish, but she tends to regard sex as a favor she gives to men rather than something primarily for her own enjoyment, even though she clearly enjoys it once she gets started. As a result, she has on several occasions since we've been married fucked with other men. She has been open about it with me, but despite her efforts at being cool, the excitement of sleeping with another man has aroused her own sexuality to the point where she becomes much more sexually awake.

As a result, the weeks following these sexual adventures have been among the most highly charged and explosive in our entire marriage. My feelings have, of course, been pretty mixed on these occasions, but on the whole, it made our fucking never better. Furthermore, I once had an affair of some duration. The only difference was that Phoebe didn't know about it until later because my lover was a close friend of ours. Anyway, fantasies have developed because I see them as the beginning of a period of enhanced sexuality between Phoebe and me.

One involves a party at our house. Phoebe is dancing closely with a particularly tall, slender man whom I've only met that evening. When the last guest leaves, they are still dancing. She looks over at me with the look of a naughty schoolgirl who knows she is misbehaving. I don't really want to spoil her fun, so I just excuse myself and go to bed. About a half hour later, I wake up and notice the music has stopped. There is a guest room with a double bed under our bedroom, and one can hear pretty well through the radiator pipes. I lean over and hear Phoebe's voice: "Oh, yes, that's nice. Please! Put it in me! I want you!" I hear more of this until finally I hear Phoebe's telltale "Uhhh, uhhhh, yes, yes, ohh!" I realize she is having a smashing climax. Then, silence. I doze off and wake up two hours later. Still, Phoebe is not in our bed. I lean over again, and I hear the now-familiar sounds just at the point of another all-out orgasm. Now I'm wide awake and hard as a rock.

About a half hour later, I hear the front door open and close, and a few minutes later, Phoebe comes sneaking into the bedroom, looking a bit disheveled but rather happy. When she realizes I am awake, she gets a somewhat sheepish look on her face, but I pull her into bed before she can go into the bathroom and wash. In an instant, my cock is in her pussy, which is juicy with another man's cum, and I have an almost instant climax. She is totally exhausted by now, and we fall asleep in each other's arms.

I told her about this fantasy, and she said she wanted to make it come true for me. I brought it up to a friend of mine that I know Phoebe is attracted to, and he was game. Going in, something told me it was a mistake. I'm not small, but his cock is huge, and with him there and Phoebe so excited, I couldn't even get hard. I felt so insignificant, a feeling I wasn't able to shake, even after it was over. It was terrible. They both had a good time, and Phoebe thought I was happy because I pretended to enjoy watching. But it didn't take her long to know something was up. I developed paranoia of not being able to satisfy her. It actually caused temporary impotency around her.

After some time and a lot of Viagra, our sex life is back on track. But I realize my fantasy of being with Phoebe and another man is just where it belongs—in fantasy.

Kenya

Kenya, a beautiful young woman who works near an Army base, had the opportunity to live out her fantasy.

When I was twenty, I'd been having a fantasy about having five or six men all to myself when suddenly it became true. I had just met Johan. We were so attracted to each other, we became instantly involved. After our first date, we made love all night.

We made plans to meet at a bar a few nights later before he went out of town, but when I got there, he was with another girl. I decided to make him jealous and fawned all over his buddies. I had one dancing hip-to-hip with me and one pressed right up against my ass, too. I also had three other guys waiting for their turn. These guys had been on exercise and were starved for girls. Johan came over and joined his friends. This went on for about an hour, me dancing with other guys, and other women chasing him around. That's when the expression "gang rape" actually took on meaning. I felt someone's hand on my arm, pulling me toward the door. Johan noticed the ruckus.

Outside, I was being stuffed in a cab. He hastily got my jacket and pursued us. He forced his way into the cab and gave words of advice. He said, "You'd better cooperate with them because they're all excited enough now that if you refuse, they'll just force you. I came because I don't want to see you hurt. I should be able to keep them from getting crazy." I started to think of my fantasy to try and enjoy it. They all came to my house, and I was full of all orifices all night. It was horrible and nothing like my fantasy of group sex.

I have four older brothers, and I used to love it when they'd play rough with me, even though they'd sometimes get in trouble for it. Maybe that's where the fantasy came from. But I always knew they'd never really hurt me. This was totally different. I wish I could have just kept it in my mind.

Sex, especially when there is only one woman and a group of men, can be a hot box that sets each man off in a different way, culminating in more than one man angry and confused at being left out—a horror of a fantasy that should have remained just that.

We are often inclined to follow our erotic fantasies as if they were real maps to a buried treasure rather than clues to who and how we are, not just sexually but beyond. Like dreams at night, our erotic reveries inform us not only of our desires but of our past. They especially open doors to who we were when very young.

I think of the world of sex not just for the pleasure it can bring but for the energy it contains, that state of well-being in which we are left post-orgasm, the brief mental balance, breathless equilibrium. Both sex and love, two very separate entities, if handled with care can be brilliant. I try to treat them with the same respect and with the same close attention I give to sharp knives and dynamite.